THE SECRET *of* ViGOR

Ordering
Trade bookstores in the U.S. and Canada please contact:

Publishers Group West
1700 Fourth Street, Berkeley CA 94710
Phone: (800) 788-3123   Fax: (800) 351-5073

Hunter House books are available at bulk discounts for textbook course adoptions; to qualifying community, health-care, and government organizations; and for special promotions and fund-raising. For details please contact:

Special Sales Department
Hunter House Inc., PO Box 2914, Alameda CA 94501-0914
Phone: (510) 865-5282   Fax: (510) 865-4295
E-mail: ordering@hunterhouse.com

Individuals can order our books from most bookstores,
by calling **(800) 266-5592**, or from our website at
www.hunterhouse.com

THE

HOW TO OVERCOME BURNOUT, RESTORE METABOLIC BALANCE

SECRET

AND RECLAIM YOUR NATURAL ENERGY

of ViGOR

Shawn M. Talbott, PhD, LDN, FACSM

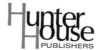

Hunter House PUBLISHERS

Hunter House Inc., Publishers
PO Box 2914
Alameda CA 94501-0914

Library of Congress Cataloging-in-Publication Data
Talbott, Shawn M.
The secret of vigor : how to overcome burnout, restore metabolic balance and reclaim your natural energy / Shawn M. Talbott.
p. cm.
ISBN 978-0-89793-573-9 (pbk.)
1. Energy metabolism. 2. Health. I. Title.
QP176.T35 2011
612.3'9--dc23
2011023473

Project Credits
Cover Design: Brian Dittmar Design, Inc.
Book Production: John McKercher and Jinni Fontana
Developmental Editors: Kelsey Comes and Mary Claire Blakeman
Copy Editor: Heather Wilcox
Proofreader: John David Marion
Indexer: Candace Hyatt
Acquisitions Assistant: Erica M. Lee
Managing Editor: Alexandra Mummery
Senior Marketing Associate: Reina Santana
Publicity and Marketing: Sean Harvey
Rights Coordinator: Candace Groskreutz
Customer Service Manager: Christina Sverdrup
Order Fulfillment: Washul Lakdhon
Administrator: Theresa Nelson
Computer Support: Peter Eichelberger
Publisher: Kiran S. Rana

Printed and bound by Sheridan Books, Ann Arbor, Michigan
Manufactured in the United States of America

9 8 7 6 5 4 3 2 1   First Edition   12 13 14 15 16

Contents

Important Note

The material in this book is intended to provide a review of information regarding the biochemical effects of stress and hormone levels on health and vigor. Every effort has been made to provide accurate and dependable information. The contents of this book have been compiled through professional research and in consultation with health professionals. However, health professionals have differing opinions, and advances in medical and scientific research are made very quickly, so some of the information may become outdated.

Therefore, the publisher, authors, and editors, as well as the professionals quoted or cited in the book, cannot be held responsible for any error, omission, or dated material. The authors and publisher assume no responsibility for any outcome of applying the information in this book in a program of self-care or under the care of a licensed practitioner. If you have questions concerning your nutrition or diet or about the application of the information described in this book, consult a qualified health-care professional.

Acknowledgments

The process of writing and revising *The Secret of Vigor* (as well as the process of conducting the numerous research studies that "prove" the approach outlined in this book) has been a constant project for me over the past six or seven years. My experiences during this period as researcher and educator have helped me refine and expand my thinking about the impact of stress and the biochemical disruptions to health and well-being that stress causes. This book — and the concept that biochemistry drives behavior — would not have been possible without the invaluable contributions over the years of the thousands of participants in my lifestyle programs and seminars. These participants were just like you in many ways: intelligent and curious people who were too busy and too stressed and were thinking that they needed to do something to get their lives (and bodies) under control. For these folks, the concepts of "Biochemical Balance" and "Vigor" provided the education and the answers they needed to regain the control they were looking for. I owe each of them a huge THANK YOU for helping me refine my thinking into the research-proven yet "real-life" approaches that you will read about in the coming pages.

I also need to thank my publisher, Kiran Rana, for believing that educating people about vigor, as this book does, is as important as simply educating people about the detrimental health effects of chronic stress, as some of my other "Cortisol Connection" books have done. Thanks also to my capable editors, Alexandra Mummery, Mary Claire Blakeman, and Heather Wilcox, who refined, streamlined, and polished the rough draft through many better and better versions — resulting in a much-more-readable and ultimately more-useful book that will truly help you realize the Secret of Vigor.

Finally, and always, I need to thank three of the major sources of vigor in my own life: my wife, Julie, and our kids, Courtney and Alexander, for their patience and understanding regarding all the work that went into *The Secret of Vigor*. Through the numerous research trials (when I'm "working"), extensive speaking tours (when I'm "away"), and constant writing (when I'm "in there" — referring to our home office), they have all granted me the "mental space" (and quiet) to refine the concepts around vigor that have helped thousands of people already and, through this book, will help many thousands more to recapture a *vigor*ous life.

Introduction

What Is Vigor?

Chances are, if you're like most other people living in any industrialized country anywhere in the world, your daily routine is hectic and stressful. You may suffer from constant fatigue, rarely sleep well, or continue to gain weight, and you're at least occasionally moody. In fact, you may be experiencing what we often refer to in psychology research as "burnout."

But what if things were different? What if you could reverse burnout — or avoid it altogether? Suppose, instead of fatigue, you felt energized? What if you enjoyed a restful eight hours of sleep every night, maintained a healthy weight, and generally stopped feeling tired, stressed, and depressed? If you achieved such a level of wellness, your condition could only be described as being the antithesis of "burnout."

This state of well-being — the opposite of burnout — has also received a name from psychology researchers: "vigor."

Outside the research community, however, very few people have heard the term "vigor" used as a measure of health. And in your own vocabulary, the word may only turn up when you're talking about *vigor*ous exercise or reading cookbook instructions that tell you to shake liquids *vigor*ously.

But "vigor" actually has an official definition in scientific circles: "a three-tiered sustained mood state characterized by physical energy, mental acuity, and emotional well-being." The chart on the next page may help you see this definition a little more clearly — and it also underscores the differences between vigor and burnout.

Vigor vs. Burnout

Vigor	Burnout
Physical energy	Physical fatigue
Mental acuity (focus)	Mental exhaustion
Cognitive Liveliness	Cognitive weariness

Vigor is a true measure of wellness, because it encompasses much more than simply feeling "energetic," having a "sharp" mind, or being in a "good mood." People with high levels of vigor are those "can-do" individuals who feel like getting things done — whether they are running a marathon or just cleaning out the garage. They're motivated and have the capacity to accomplish what they set out to do, because they're not weighed down by feeling sleep deprived or exhausted all the time. Unfortunately, for a lot of people, "vigor" is a state that they have not experienced in many years, but that does not mean they cannot reclaim it. These are the people I wrote this book for — because I know from my research and experience with countless clients that people can build and maintain the vigor that may be missing in their lives.

THE SECRET OF VIGOR: BIOCHEMICAL BALANCE

When it comes to improving your well-being, you often hear limited "one-dimensional" advice that focuses on a single aspect of health. You know: "...eat this super-food!" "...do this special exercise!" "...take this pill!" Many aspects of Western medicine, in fact, address isolated symptoms instead of the overall condition of your body. To understand how to improve your level of vigor, it is important to appreciate the intricacies of the human body as a whole system. Biochemistry can help you gain this appreciation, because it is, essentially, the study of those intricacies — the processes going on within your body that make it possible for you to live. And, crucially, your biochemistry holds the key to your level of vigor.

To get a better idea of what I'm talking about, take a moment to imagine the most complicated, beautiful machine that you can think of. Did you envision a supercomputer? An automobile? A satellite? The International Space Station? Certainly, these are all very complex machines, and perhaps they're even beautiful from an engineering point of view. But their complexity pales in comparison to that of the human body. The body is a dynamic, ever-changing, always-adapting collection of intricate structures and systems. Sometimes it works perfectly on its own — your lungs fill and empty, your heart beats, and your eyes blink — all without your having to remember to "work" them. But sometimes your body breaks down. In most circumstances, the damage is only tempo-rary, because your internal repair mechanisms jump into action to fix the damage and get you back to full function. Sometimes, how-ever, the damage persists. You accumulate little bits of damage and dings and creaks over the years, and you find yourself waking up one morning with physical ailments, such an aching knee, a stiff back, or a generalized pain through your entire body. Sometimes the ailments are more "psychological" in nature, such as depres-sion, fatigue, brain fog, lack of motivation, or outright burnout.

Whether physical or mental, all these ailments have their roots in problems with the biochemistry of your body. Specifically, I'm referring to the biochemical activity among hormones, blood-sugar levels, brain signals, and the other internal interactions that take place below the surface of your skin that you are hardly aware of — until something goes wrong. When the balance between hor-mones, such as cortisol and testosterone, or between neurotrans-mitters, such as dopamine and norepinephrine, is disrupted, you can be left feeling "blah" or even burned out. If internal imbalances lead to burnout, then reestablishing biochemical balance has the opposite effect — it produces vigor.

Quite simply, the "secret" of vigor is to balance your biochemistry.

Or, as I sometimes say to people who want a simple way to remember this idea: Balance your biochemistry to beat burnout!

In my years of research on this subject, I have found four basic biochemical processes that need to be brought into balance for anyone who wants to improve their health and vigor. I've labeled these processes the "Four Pillars of Health." Let's take a brief look at them.

THE FOUR PILLARS OF HEALTH

When you tap the secret of vigor, you're not just making short-term cosmetic changes to your sense of well-being — you're uncovering the root causes of exhaustion and excess stress hidden in the biochemistry of your cells. The best way to balance your biochemistry is to strengthen the "Four Pillars of Health": manage oxidation, control inflammation, stabilize glucose, and balance stress hormones. Here's a list of these pillars for your quick reference:

The Four Pillars of Health

1. manage oxidation
2. control inflammation
3. stabilize glucose
4. balance stress hormones

Each of the Four Pillars of Health describes rather complicated biochemical processes that are explained in more detail in Part II of this book. For now, the important thing to understand is that you need balance within and among these four processes to develop and maintain vigor.

Vigor in Ancient Medicine

Besides recognizing the role of your biochemistry in the pursuit of health, it can also be helpful to have another way to think about vigor, because the term "vigor," as used in psychology research today, actually has very old roots. The modern scientific concept of vigor is somewhat comparable to the ancient descriptions of vitality and wellness from traditional medicine systems around the world. Nearly every ancient culture has typically held a common belief that true health stems from a strong "life force" in the body. Other names for this life force, or vigor, include:

- *qi* (traditional Chinese medicine; pronounced "chee")
- *ki* (Kampo/Japanese medicine)
- *prana* (Ayurvedic/Indian medicine)
- *ka* (Egyptian medicine)
- *mana* (Polynesian medicine)
- *pneuma* (ancient Greek medicine)

Practitioners of traditional medicine might have restored "life force" in their patients by improving their nutrition or administering herbal medicines. These natural therapies often "worked," and patients felt better as a result. What these ancient healers did not fully appreciate was "how" their therapies were working to actually alter biochemical processes in the body and modulate the internal interactions that I'm calling the Four Pillars of Health.

In modern times, millions of people attempt to temporarily reduce fatigue with energy drinks or other stimulants. However, that approach does not restore vigor and is actually more likely to sap vigor in the long term. These temporary "fixes" are inadequate solutions, because they do not address the underlying cause of low vigor: biochemical imbalances between and among the Four Pillars. Although this book highlights current research on vigor and health, it also incorporates the guiding principle of traditional medicines—that true wellness results from a comprehensive, balanced view of the human body, not one that focuses on fragmented, short-term "fixes."

VALIDATING VIGOR:
PROFILE OF MOOD STATES (POMS)

As you continue reading, one key concept you will discover is that chronic stress has a significant impact on your level of vigor. Chronic stress — and the underlying biochemical imbalances that it leads to — undoubtedly plays a major role in many of today's modern diseases, particularly depression, chronic fatigue, anxiety, fibromyalgia, and obesity. In fact, according to the Centers for Disease Control and Prevention and the World Health Organization:

- 80 percent of North Americans have enough daily stress to cause health problems.
- Stress contributes to half of all illnesses in North America.
- 70–80 percent of all doctor visits are for stress-related illnesses.
- More than half of all deaths in people under the age of sixty-five result from stressful lifestyles.

The good news is that by naturally restoring biochemical balance, you can dramatically reduce feelings of stress, cut fatigue and depression, boost physical and mental energy, and significantly improve vigor.

How can I make these claims about improving vigor? Because, in labs and clinics, researchers can actually measure vigor using a scientifically validated research tool called the Profile of Mood States (POMS) questionnaire.

The POMS is a psychological rating system that measures specific transitory moods in a variety of populations, including medical patients, psychiatric outpatients, and athletes, among other fields. It has been used in more than three thousand research studies, making it the true "gold standard" for assessing changes in mood state and vigor following different interventions (such as exercise programs, nutritional regimens, stress-reduction techniques, and intake of dietary supplements).

The POMS assesses six primary psychological factors — tension, depression, anger, fatigue, vigor, and confusion — by asking sixty-five adjective-based questions scored on a "0–4" intensity scale (with intensity being gauged as 0 = not at all and 4 = extremely). The sixty-five adjective responses are categorized into the six psychological factors, tabulated, scored, and analyzed. The output of the POMS questionnaire is an assessment of the positive and negative moods of each subject at baseline and at various intervals throughout the study intervention (typically four, eight, and twelve weeks later).

Over the past several years, my research group has conducted a series of human clinical studies in "stressed" volunteers. In these studies — some as short as one week and others as long as twelve weeks — we have been able to significantly improve vigor by 25 to 30 percent following a restoration of biochemical balance. This means that, although chronic stress *disrupts* biochemical balance, we now know that *restoring* biochemical balance can help improve feelings of vigor quickly (sometimes within the first week of the study period). We've also found that these changes persist for months thereafter, indicating a unique and lasting improvement in overall well-being that is far superior to the temporary effects of energy drinks and related products. These clinical trials have been presented at some of the top peer-reviewed scientific conferences in the world, including the American College of Nutrition, American College of Sports Medicine, the International Society for Sports Nutrition, and the American Society for Nutrition.

It may be hard to understand how something as simple as stress can cause so many problems — from depression to heart disease to weight gain. But the fact is, your body's response to everyday pressures — including deadlines, traffic, money concerns, family conflicts, irritating coworkers, and other worries — is actually a chronic-stress response. And that response to chronic stress causes an immediate and profound change in a variety of hormones and related biochemicals in your body. Further, those compounds are distributed throughout the entire body, where they influence the function of every organ and cell.

Initially, the effects of chronic stress are subtle. On the hormonal level, cortisol goes up, and testosterone goes down. Although you are hardly likely to detect such hormonal changes on a daily basis, what you might notice is that you experience a few extra pounds of weight, a slight reduction in energy levels, a modest drop in sex drive, or a bit of trouble with memory. Even then, you probably brush off these health signals as "normal" aspects of aging. However, as you'll read in *The Secret of Vigor*, these traits are actually the earliest signs of depression, chronic fatigue, fibromyalgia, obesity, diabetes, impotence, dementia, heart disease, cancer, and many related conditions — and chronic stress can trigger all of them. Indeed, researchers are discovering that stress may well be the key factor in the very process commonly recognized as "aging."

Still, it can be hard to accept the idea that the stress you go through every day can have such a detrimental effect on your long-term health as well as your daily level of vigor. But once you understand the relationship between modern stressors and your biochemical balance, I am certain that you will be *motivated to do something* about getting your biochemistry back into balance.

But first, let's see where you stand in terms of vigor and wellness right now. You can check your exposure to stress — and your risk for falling into the trap of unbalanced biochemistry and low vigor — with a simple questionnaire called the "Vigor Self-Test." Because it can be very difficult to recognize the telltale signs associated with stress-induced health problems, such as those described in the preceding few paragraphs, this test can help gauge your overall exposure to stress. The "Vigor Self-Test" presented below is a version of the standard POMS test used for assessing vigor in countless studies. My research group has also used this questionnaire for several years to measure stress levels and the degree of biochemical balance or imbalance in the people who participate in our studies.

The Vigor Self-Test

- For each question, write your score in the corresponding column.
- For each answer of "Never/No"—give yourself zero (0) points.
- For each answer of "Occasionally"—give yourself one (1) point.
- For each answer of "Frequently/Yes"—give yourself two (2) points.
- For the last question (#16)—SUBTRACT 1 point for each of the words that closely describes how you have been feeling during the past TWO WEEKS.

Question—"How Often Do You..."

1. ...experience stressful situations?   _____

2. ...feel tired or fatigued?   _____

3. ...get fewer than eight hours of sleep?   _____

4. ...feel anxious/depressed?   _____

5. ...feel overwhelmed or confused?   _____

6. ...have a low sex drive?   _____

7. ...put on weight around the belly?   _____

8. ...diet to lose weight?   _____

9. ...attempt to control your body weight?   _____

10. ...pay close attention to the foods you eat?   _____

11. ...crave carbohydrates (sweets or breads)?   _____

12. ...experience problems concentrating?   _____

13. ...experience tension headaches?   _____

14. ...experience digestive problems or heartburn?   _____

15. ...get sick or catch colds/flu?   _____

Scoring (add above numbers #1–#15)   **points** _____

16. ...feel lively, active, energetic, cheerful, alert, full of pep, carefree, or vigorous (one point for each, 0–8 total)?   _____

Total (subtract total for #16 from total for #1–#15)   **points** _____

Vigor Index

0–5 points   **High Vigor** (Excellent Biochemical Balance)
You are cool as a cucumber and have either a very low level of stress
or a tremendous ability to deal effectively with incoming stressors.
Keep doing what you're doing!

6–10 points   **Average Vigor** (Acceptable Biochemical Balance)
You may be suffering from an overexposure to stress or an overactive stress response, and you are at moderate risk of being chronically out of biochemical balance, leading to reduced vigor. You should
incorporate anti-stress strategies into your lifestyle whenever possible to maintain (and improve) your biochemical balance and vigor.
But don't stress out about it!

Greater than 10 points   **Low Vigor** (OUT of Biochemical Balance)
The bad news is that you're almost definitely suffering from an overactive stress response, chronically disrupted biochemical balance,
and a low state of vigor—and you need to take immediate steps to
regain control. The good news is that you're not alone—literally millions of people are in the same situation.

If your test results show you have a low vigor score, you are not
going to keel over tomorrow from a lack of biochemical balance —
nor does it mean that the rare person with a high vigor score will
necessarily live to a ripe old age. In reality, virtually anyone who
experiences stress on a regular basis, gets fewer than eight hours of
sleep each night, or is simply aging is on the fast track to being out
of biochemical balance. Therefore, everyone can benefit from targeted steps to maintain or restore their biochemical balance and to
improve their personal levels of vigor. In times of particularly high
stress — such as when you're moving, switching jobs, or undergoing changes in close relationships — you will need to focus more
carefully on efforts to boost your vigor. At other times, when you
have less stress in your life — perhaps during a vacation — your attention to biochemical balance can wander a bit.

Ultimately, the reality is that living in the twenty-first century yields a certain amount of unavoidable stress. With that stress come disruptions in your biochemistry, such as elevations in levels of the hormone cortisol accompanied by suppressed testosterone levels. This means that the choices you make in how you *deal* with stress and the things you do to *balance* your biochemistry can make a critical difference in terms of your long-term health and the way you feel on a daily basis. So keep reading. Whatever your score on the Vigor Self-Test, this book has been written to help you improve your overall health — and feel better while you're doing it.

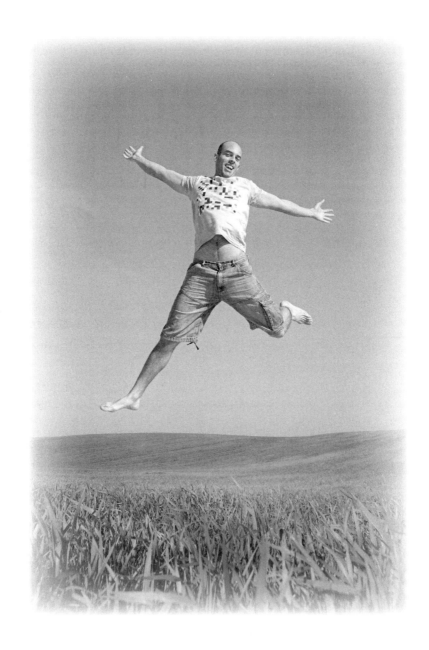

PART I *The Science of Vigor*

If the secret of vigor is to balance the biochemistry of your body to beat burnout, then you need to know a little about how that biochemistry works. Don't worry, you won't need to memorize complex anatomy charts or chemical formulas. Instead, if you simply understand a few key insights about the vital processes that occur within your body, you will be armed with the knowledge you need to become healthier and happier. These insights provide the foundation for what I call the "science of vigor."

One of the fundamental biochemical facts you need to know is this: Chronic stress robs you of vigor. The unrelenting, chronic stress that most people put up with every day can wreak havoc with their sleep, weight, and general health — and it can also lead to serious medical problems, ranging from diabetes and osteoporosis to cancer and heart disease. In Chapter 1, you'll find out some of the ways stress affects the body — and why stress is the nemesis of vigor.

Your biochemistry affects you not only physically but mentally and emotionally as well. In fact, the second key insight in the science of vigor is this: Biochemistry drives emotions — and behavior. Not only that, but your brain chemistry also affects your actions to a much greater degree than has ever been recognized before. Chapter 2 covers all these issues.

13

After reading about the basics of biochemistry in Part I, you'll be ready to drill down a little deeper into the hidden chemistry taking place on the cellular level of your body. These biochemical activities — the Four Pillars of Health — are the focus of Part II.

Finally, in Part III, you'll discover how you can apply these concepts about biochemistry to your own daily life by engaging in Vigor Improvement Practices — and that is where you will find the real value of the science of vigor.

1

Chronic Stress —
The Enemy of Vigor

onventional wisdom and countless commercials bombard us with the idea that the way to get healthy is simply to exercise more and eat a better diet. Both these habits are certainly important parts of being healthy, but from my perspective as a biochemist, I'm going to tell you something you'll hardly hear from anyone else: If you truly want to improve your health, *it is just as important to get your stress levels under control as it is to eat a healthy diet and to get physical activity*! Quite simply, stress has a bigger impact on your life and well-being than almost anything else you encounter. Most people don't understand this fact, or else they ignore it. Worse, some people think they're "tough" enough to handle all the stress in their lives. Nothing could be farther from the truth, because stress sets off major biochemical changes in the body. And that is why I call stress the number-one enemy of vigor.

The stressed-out feeling that many people experience may seem "typical," simply because everyone else is experiencing it, too. But that does not mean it is "normal" in a physiological sense, nor is it an indicator of good health or well-being. The body, including the nervous system and endocrine (hormonal) system, was simply not meant for the chronic stress that people face as part of their everyday lives in the twenty-first century. Most people simply endure this "twenty-first-century syndrome," that familiar feeling of always being "on," of being rushed, harried, and frantic. That is what chronic stress feels like, and it leads to a state of low vigor or "burnout," with its accompanying fatigue, depression, and mental fog.

As just one indication that chronic stress is taking a toll on the populace, consider this: The incidence of depression and anxiety in modern society is now ten times higher than it was just a generation ago. Some researchers attribute this staggering increase to physicians' diagnosing psychological "diseases" at a higher rate, because they now have drugs to "cure" them. But it could also be due to the fact that many people are simply living lives that feel constantly out of control. Not only are levels of depression and anxiety on the rise, but close to ninety million cases of diseases with "no known cause" have been diagnosed. These diseases range from chronic fatigue syndrome (CFS), fibromyalgia (FM), vital exhaustion ("burnout"), and irritable bowel syndrome (IBS) to recurrent yeast infections, autoimmune disease, chronic back pain, and other "nonspecific" conditions. The never-ending stress under which people toil on a daily basis plays a role in all these illnesses and conditions, yet Western doctors and researchers are often slow to admit that "mental" conditions, such as stress, can have physical effects upon the rest of the body. They fail to recognize that stress, which leads to biochemical imbalances, is the underlying cause of poor health and low vigor.

Because your ability to improve your vigor is so intricately connected to the way you deal with stress, I want to give you a brief tutorial on this subject. Readers interested in a more detailed overview of the relationship between stress and disease may want to refer to my previous book, *The Cortisol Connection,* 2nd edition (Hunter House Publishers). Let's begin with a quick look at the definition of stress.

STRESS—WHAT IS IT, REALLY?

A simple way to understand the meaning of stress is to define it as "what you feel when life's demands exceed your ability to meet those demands." Every individual, of course, has a different capacity to effectively cope with stress and a different level of functioning when faced with stressful situations. Everyone knows people who function better "under pressure" than others. But even the rare person who has a high tolerance for stress ultimately has a breaking point. Add enough total stress to anyone, and both health and performance inevitably suffer.

To deepen your understanding of stress, it is helpful to recognize the distinctions that many of the top stress researchers in the world use when analyzing this condition. First is the type of stress faced by your cousins in the animal kingdom, which are short-term, temporary, or *acute* stressors. That sort of stress is distinct from the type of stressors that modern humans routinely face, because our stressors are longer-term, repeated, and *chronic*. In addition, unlike animals, humans undergo not only physical stress but also psychological and social stress. Certainly, some sources of psychological stress are grounded in reality, such as the pressure you feel to make your monthly rent or mortgage payments. Other psychological stressors emanate from your imagination—for instance, the stressful encounters that you can imagine having with your boss, coworkers, kids, spouse, or others. So not only do you have to cope with real-life stressors, but your large, complex, and supposedly "advanced" brain has also developed the capacity to actually *create* stressful situations where none previously existed.

THE BIOCHEMISTRY OF STRESS

In research circles, the response of a zebra facing a possible attack by a lion is used as a standard example to explain stress physiology. In this example, the zebra represents you, and the lion represents your stress. If you were to face a charging lion, your body would quickly pace itself through a series of neurological, biochemical, hormonal, and physiological actions. These actions are labeled with a term you've probably heard: the "fight-or-flight" response. Each response mechanism within your body is designed to help you run away from the lion — that is, to take flight — or engage it in battle — to fight (and, you hope, to survive for another day).

For zebras, the stress response runs its complete course, from start to finish, in a relatively short period of time. When the zebra experiences a stressor, such as the lion charging, its brain and hormone system release a series of stress hormones. This stress response enables the zebra to fight off the lion or run away from it. That is the classic "fight-or-flight" response. After getting away from the lion, the zebra's stress hormones return to normal. The zebra goes on to live happily and healthily ever after — at least until the next lion shows up. Most importantly, the entire process, from the point when the zebra sees the lion until its hormones return to normal, takes perhaps sixty seconds from start to finish. This short episode, and the zebra's response to it, is a perfect example of what researchers refer to as "acute stress" or "temporary stress." This is the type of stress that gets you up and going and to which you can adapt very nicely because it is over so quickly. Think about jumping out of the way of a bicyclist while walking in the city or dropping a cooking spoon that has become too hot from sitting next to the stove — these are examples of "temporary-stress" responses, because your body quickly reacts and just as quickly recovers.

Unfortunately for humans, many of the things that cause stress today are hard to fight off and almost impossible to run away from — unlike the zebra who can flee from the lion. Stressors come in the form of monthly mortgage payments, credit-card bills, project deadlines, traffic jams, family commitments, and myriad other pressures. Worse, these stressors seem to keep coming back again and again, making them anything but "acute," temporary, or short-term in nature. As a result, many people are in the position of being chronically "stuck" midway through the normal, temporary-stress response cycle. Because this response cycle does not have an opportunity to run its course to a natural conclusion (as it does for the zebra), people's stress hormones remain continuously elevated. The ongoing elevation of these hormones slowly leads people down the path to low vigor and toward poor long-term health.

What happens to the biochemistry of your body when you experience stress? Essentially, stress makes your cortisol levels go up. And just what is cortisol? Cortisol is a steroid hormone produced in the adrenal glands in response to stress. It is often called the primary "stress hormone," but it also shows up under the names "cortisone" or "hydrocortisone." Cortisol, basically, allows the body to maintain normal physiological processes during times of stress. In other words, without cortisol, the body would be incapable of dealing with stress effectively. Without cortisol, that lion charging at you from the bushes would cause you to do little more than to wet your pants and stand there staring. By contrast, when the body metabolizes cortisol effectively, you're primed to run away or to do battle, because cortisol secretion releases amino acids (from muscle), glucose (from the liver), and fatty acids (from adipose tissue) into the bloodstream for use as energy. Given these benefits, it might seem safe to assume that cortisol is "good" — right? The answer is yes — and no.

On the plus side, not only does the body produce cortisol to help people respond to stress, but synthetic forms of this hormone (such as prednisone and dexamethasone) are also used to treat a wide variety of conditions because of their anti-inflammatory and immune-suppressing properties. In addition, anyone who has dealt with poison ivy or similar conditions knows that cortisol-like drugs can be quite helpful in relieving the itching or excessive inflammation that accompanies certain skin disorders. These drugs are also useful during organ transplantation and in the treatment of inflammatory diseases, such as arthritis, colitis, or asthma.

And for people with Addison's disease who have lost function of their adrenal glands, cortisol-like drugs play a role in replacement-therapy regimens.

So, again, it would seem that cortisol is a "good thing" — right? Yes, but only at certain levels and for a certain period of time. When your body produces too much cortisol for too long a period of time, this can affect your health in negative ways and leave you in a situation where stress eventually leads to feeling "stressed out," which then leads to low vigor and burnout.

"STRESSED OUT"— THE DOWNSIDE OF CHRONIC STRESS

When people reach a breaking point in the face of too many pressures and worries, it is common to hear them say they are "stressed out." People usually have a sense of what those words mean, but it is important to understand the difference between being simply "stressed" and being "stressed *out*." When you are "stressed," your body undergoes an *adaptive* response. Cortisol goes up and then it comes down, as described in the example of the zebra. Being "stressed *out*" suggests that your body is unable to mount a normal stress response. If you are "stressed out," your cortisol rhythm stays flat — which means that your overall cortisol exposure over a twenty-four hour period is actually higher, because you never get a break from it. This unrelenting, "maladaptive" cortisol response is the hallmark of being "stressed out" — a condition that results from chronic stress.

The bad news is that modern society makes chronic stress largely inescapable. In research studies, scientists at Ohio University have shown that overall exposure to cortisol is significantly related to the degree of "daily hassles" (more hassles = more cortisol) as well as to age (higher age = higher cortisol) and to hours slept (less sleep = more cortisol). Worse than that, being "stressed out" (that is, coping with chronic stress) is believed to be the cause of many common diseases, such as chronic fatigue, fibromyalgia, post-traumatic stress disorder (PTSD), depression, and burnout, according to scientists at Rockefeller University in New York. And researchers in Boston have suggested that chronic psychological stress is a primary cause not just of cortisol overexposure but also of inflammatory diseases, including insulin resistance, diabetes, obesity, and heart disease.

When it comes to managing your weight or combating obesity, you also have to seriously consider the impact of the cortisol overexposure that accompanies chronic stress. To begin with, the level of inflammation in your body and the accumulation of abdominal fat (belly fat) are inextricably linked. That link takes place because cortisol and cytokines promote fat storage in a "chicken-and-egg" scenario in which it is often hard to tell which came first — the stress (which causes an overexposure to cortisol) or the inflammation (altered by the cytokines). (Cytokines, explained in more detail in Part II, are a class of hormonelike signaling proteins that play a central role in the immune response and in the level of inflammation found throughout the body.) On the cellular level, inflammation leads to obesity, which leads to more stress and inflammation, which leads to more obesity. On the other side of the coin, reducing obesity has the opposite effect: Weight loss leads to a substantial drop in inflammation and cortisol levels. And controlling stress can lead weight loss. So the "chicken-and-egg" scenario that plays out between stress-related cortisol overexposure and cytokine-regulated levels of inflammation can run two ways, positively as well as negatively. When cortisol and cytokines are locked in a downward spiral, more inflammation and more obesity result; and when that cycle is reversed, people experience weight loss. As you can see here and as you will learn throughout this book, it is the ability to manage chronic stress that determines whether these biochemical cycles turn in the right direction.

HOW CHRONIC STRESS SABOTAGES SLEEP
AND SAPS YOUR VIGOR

Have you ever had the experience of being exhausted during the day and all you can think about is getting some sleep? And then, when your head finally hits the pillow, you're wide awake! Logically this "dynamic duo" of fatigue plus insomnia (or night-time restlessness) would seem to be opposites: If you're so tired, why can't you fall asleep? However, these conditions are commonly found together in the two-thirds of the North American population who report experiencing chronic stress and who also get inadequate sleep. The common element? You guessed it: disruptions in the body's biochemical balance. That imbalance is characterized by too much cortisol, too little testosterone, and the cascade of metabolic disruptions that ensue.

In the previous section, I discussed what happens when stress-induced imbalances in cortisol and cytokines precipitate a downward spiral that leads to obesity. By the same token, the combination of fatigue and insomnia also sets off a vicious cycle in which stress makes it hard to relax and to fall asleep — which then leads to more fatigue. And being more fatigued after a sleepless night makes it harder to deal with stressors, which then causes even *more* difficulty falling asleep the next night…and the next night and the next after that in a repetitive cycle that ultimately ends in burnout.

Now you can begin to see how all these stress-driven disruptions to the hidden biochemistry within your body can have a real impact on your health, sabotaging your sleep and sapping your vigor. But how does biochemical balance fit into this picture? As you've learned in this chapter, stress induces a rise in cortisol-exposure levels. And one of the many effects of cortisol is to increase your level of alertness, which means that encountering stressful events in the late afternoon or early evening will cause your body to go "on alert," much the way a zebra would jump at the sound of an approaching lion. That spike in your alertness then hampers your ability to relax and fall asleep at night. On top of that, if you don't get to bed at a reasonable hour — early enough to allow a full eight hours of shut-eye — your cortisol metabolism doesn't get a chance to completely "step through" its normal rhythm pattern. Within this normal pattern, cortisol levels reach their lowest point around 3:00 AM. As a result, you may get only five, six, or seven hours of sleep and wake up feeling groggy after having been exposed to higher-than-normal levels of cortisol throughout the night.

Once cortisol hits bottom around 3:00 AM, it tends to rise again and normally peaks in the early morning, from about 6:00 AM to 8:00 AM. If you think about it, that makes perfect sense, because cortisol increases your alertness. So your body's cortisol levels rise in the early morning as a way to get you moving and prepared to face the challenges of the day. Then, as the morning wears on, between the hours of 8:00 AM and 11:00 AM, cortisol levels begin to drop and gradually decline throughout the day. That decline in cortisol typically causes you to feel a decrease in your energy level and ability to concentrate sometime around 3:00 PM to 4:00 PM. Office workers and others often call this the "afternoon slump." This dip in energy levels is the body's way of saying, "The day is almost over; better get ready for sleep." Instead of getting ready for sleep, however, modern lifestyles cause most people to look for ways to boost their energy levels late in the day so they can get through afternoon meetings, soccer practices, piano recitals, business dinners, and time with their families. The average body clock really wants you to eat your last meal of the day around 5:00 PM and to be asleep by 8:00 PM. Unfortunately, wristwatches, television sets, computers, video games, and other electronics often keep you awake late into the night.

In the long run, when you sleep fewer hours than the recommended standard eight hours per night, you can experience annoying side effects, such as headaches, irritability, frequent infections, depression, anxiety, confusion, and generalized mental and physical fatigue. Not only can the lack of sleep leave you feeling lousy and low on vigor, but research shows that even mild sleep deprivation can actually destroy a person's long-term health and increase the risk of burnout, diabetes, obesity, and breast cancer. *In many ways, sleeping fewer than eight hours each night is as bad for overall wellness as gorging on junk food or becoming a couch potato!*

On the biochemical level, one of the major problems with the modern "late to bed, early to rise" lifestyle is that your cortisol levels never have enough time to fully dissipate as they are supposed to do during the overnight resting period. As a result, your body never has a chance to fully recover and repair itself from the detrimental effects of chronic stress. That overexposure to cortisol throws a "monkey wrench" into your ability to maintain biochemical balance. And when your biochemical balance is out of whack, it sends your overall metabolism into a downward spiral, accelerating the "breakdown" of tissues and sending your energy, mood, and mental focus into a tailspin, leaving you with low vigor.

BALANCING BIOCHEMISTRY AND BUILDING VIGOR

When measuring the state of their health through lab tests, people often want to bring their "numbers" down. For instance, they may strive to *lower* their cholesterol or to *lower* high blood-pressure readings. But when it comes to the subject of stress, the goal is not simply to *lower* cortisol levels. In fact, many stress physiologists believe that it is not the *absolute* level of cortisol people are exposed to but their degrees of cortisol *variability* that indicate a healthy stress response. In other words, people should aim to have neither high cortisol nor low cortisol but instead a cortisol level that *fluctuates* normally in response to stress and relaxation. Chronically high cortisol is bad, and chronically low cortisol is also bad — but "flat" levels that show little to no fluctuation seem to be just as bad as either extreme, because they lead to problems with biochemical balance and to adverse changes in other hormones farther "down-stream" in the metabolic cascade.

Ideally, cortisol levels should rise and fall in a rhythm that is responsive and variable. That variability means cortisol levels should remain low at night and when you are relaxed, but climb during periods of acute stress, exercise, and work deadlines, recovering to lower baseline levels quickly. We do not want cortisol to stay at any one level "chronically," whether high, low, or medium. Rather, we want cortisol *flux*. We want a highly responsive, finely tuned pattern of cortisol activity. In stress research, then, the emphasis on measuring whether cortisol levels are "high" or "low" has shifted. Instead, researchers want to know how those levels *fluctuate* over time, how they are balanced with other aspects of biochemistry, and what people's overall twenty-four-hour exposure may be to cortisol and to a growing collection of other hormones, enzymes, cytokines, and neurotransmitters.

The importance of having fluctuating cortisol levels cannot be overstated. In fact, a pattern of "flat" cortisol rhythm is one indicator of stress overload. A "flat" reading means that cortisol levels may be within ranges that might be labeled "normal," but they do not appear to increase in response to stress or to fall during periods of relaxation. As a result, the body is constantly exposed to "moderate" levels of cortisol on a twenty-four-hour basis. Such exposures can lead to the worst-case scenarios for long-term health. For example, people with chronic-stress diseases, such as vital exhaustion (burnout), chronic fatigue syndrome, and fibromyalgia, are known to exhibit a "flat" cortisol rhythm, as are sufferers of PTSD (post-traumatic stress disorder) and children who have suffered physical abuse. According to German researchers, when cortisol rhythms become flattened, an enzyme inside abdominal fat cells (called "HSD," for hydroxy-steroid-dehydrogenase) kicks into overdrive to increase cortisol levels—and cortisol is a potent trigger for fat storage in those same belly-fat cells. As you can imagine, when the HSD increases cortisol levels, the cortisol, in turn, increases fat storage in the belly. And all that hormonal activity takes place in the abdominal region, even if the rest of the body contains cortisol in the "normal" range.

When chronic stress disrupts your healthy fluctuation of cortisol levels, it often leaves you feeling fatigued during the day (when you should feel energized) and restless at night (when you want to be relaxed). A "flattened" cortisol rhythm also sets off a cascade of detrimental alterations in other aspects of biochemical balance, including elevations in oxidative free radicals, inflammatory cytokines, and sugars associated with glycation (all covered in more detail in Part II).

VALUING VIGOR

You've just learned a great deal about biochemistry, and at this point you may have a better understanding of how the hormone cortisol affects your body. You may also have come to realize that chronic stress is not only a major stumbling block to developing daily vigor but a threat to your long-term health as well. It is my hope that, as you continue reading, you will recognize vigor as a quality to be valued, cherished, and cultivated.

2

Biochemistry Drives Emotions — and Behaviors

In seeking to build vigor, it is important to remember that this state of health is characterized not only by physical energy but also by mental acuity and emotional well-being, as you learned in the Introduction. Because the last chapter explains the physical effects of stress, it is now time to look at the emotional and mental aspects of vigor.

When speaking before thousands of people around the country, one of the most important concepts that I try to convey to my audiences is that "biochemistry drives emotions" and vice-versa. The reason that you "feel" a certain way is because of your underlying biochemistry. The degree to which you're exposed to cortisol, dopamine, serotonin, insulin, or hundreds of other "signals" in the body will influence your feelings of energy, happiness, mental clarity, creativity, appetite, and motivation — in short, your vigor. Think about how you feel when you're under stress: You often eat more (and eat more junk) and exercise less. You tend to be constantly tired during the day and yet can't relax enough to get a good night's sleep. Stressed-out people also have more heart attacks, more depression, more colds, and less sex. And stress-induced disruptions in their internal biochemistry are at the root of it all. I cannot think of a more dismal picture.

BRAINS, BIOCHEMISTRY, AND BEHAVIOR

As I have continued my research in this area over the past several years, I have discovered that the influence of biochemistry goes far deeper than ever imagined. In fact, biochemistry not only drives emotions but motivates actions as well! Breakthroughs in brain research are providing amazing new insights about these connections between biochemistry, the brain, and behavior. And, frankly, this is a complex issue that may be hard to understand. It can be mind-boggling — literally — to realize that your *thinking* can change not only your moods but also *the actual shape and function* of your brain. Those changes affect your biochemistry and, of course, your vigor.

As you read this chapter, these complex concepts will become clearer. For now, let me give you a brief explanation and illustration to show you how these mind-body-biochemistry connections work. First, you have to conceptualize the biochemical processes of your body as a circular loop, not a straight, linear progression. What happens internally is that your biochemistry affects your brain circuitry, which affects your behavior, with each influencing and feeding back on each other. This loop has no "start" and no "end," and each process constantly modifies the others. Here's what it looks like:

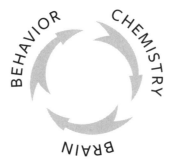

Figure 2.1. Brain circuitry—the link between biochemistry and behavior.

What does this mean in terms of building your vigor? The answer can be as perplexing as a Zen koan. Is low vigor a "biochemical" issue, a "behavioral" issue, or a "brain" issue? Yes, yes, and yes! As you've seen above, each of these issues affects the others.

The good news is that if you change one aspect of this picture, you'll inevitably change the others as well. For example, if you change your behavior — say you begin to take short walks every day or go to sleep fifteen minutes earlier each night — you will, in turn, change your biochemistry and your brain. Those brain alterations will put you into a mental and emotional state where you will want to continue the behaviors that are creating the positive mood and mental clarity — and the changes in your biochemistry will, in turn, reinforce this "virtuous circle."

Unfortunately, the "circle" can spin in the opposite direction as well. Suppose that instead of walking every day, you act like a "couch potato," sitting on the sofa watching TV for long stretches and eating greasy, sugary foods? That behavior will lead toward fatigue, mental sluggishness, and negative emotions. As your behavior begins having detrimental effects on your brain function and biochemistry, a downward spiral toward burnout is set into motion.

If you feel caught in that downward spiral, keep in mind that you are not the only one. Keep reading.

LOW VIGOR AND HIGH STRESS? YOU'RE NOT ALONE

Do you ever feel that you're working harder and harder but still getting further and further behind? If so, you have a lot of company. The average American workweek, research shows, has mushroomed from forty hours to fifty hours in the past twenty-five years. That level is higher than in any European country and equal to that of Japan. Those extra ten hours of work, however, have not gained workers much. In fact, U.S. workers today are *behind* in their ability to maintain the same overall standard of living enjoyed a generation ago. At the same time, their expectations have not changed. Even during tough economic times, people still feel pressure to be — or have — the best, whether they strive to own the best car or house or to be the best worker or parent. Talk about stress! And all those expectations are driving many to an early burnout. It is even becoming evident in kids, who run from school or day care to the babysitter to soccer to homework at the same frantic pace. Is it any wonder that the use of Ritalin and Prozac among North American children has increased, as has the diagnosis of ADHD (attention-deficit hyperactivity disorder)?

Consider this too: When the American Psychological Association (APA) released its annual 2010 survey *Stress in America,* it showed that the picture of an "overstressed nation" is as bad as it has ever been. One of the most striking conclusions from the APA survey was that "stress is not only taking a toll on our personal and physical health, but it is also affecting the emotional and physical well-being of children and our families." The survey highlighted the fact that children today are more stressed than in years past and also found that kids easily recognize and identify their parents' stress levels as a key source of their own stress.

As you might imagine, the most common sources of stress identified in the APA survey were money (76 percent), work (70 percent), and the economy (65 percent). But "family responsibilities" also emerged as a significant source of stress (73 percent).

Health experts identify a "healthy stress level" at about a 3 to 4 on a 10-point scale, with 1 representing low stress and 10 indicating extreme stress. Healthy *intermittent* exposure to stress can actually be a good thing. Some stress researchers, including myself, refer to this intermittent or "temporary" stress as "eustress" — that is, the type of stress that helps motivate you to meet a deadline or to achieve a goal. But *chronic* stress (or "distress") leads to problems with biochemical balance, tissue breakdown, and a wide range of physical and psychological health problems that result in low vigor.

The average stress level reported in the APA survey was 5.5, with 24 percent reporting stress levels at 8 to 10 (on the 10-point scale). Those with "more stress" (average of 6.2) tended to have "fair/poor" overall health, while those with "lower stress" (average of 4.9) tended to have "very good/excellent" health statuses. Individuals with even higher stress exposure (in the 8 to 10 range) tended to have significant problems with their weight or even obesity — very likely due to problems with biochemical balance and especially to an overexposure to cortisol and its associated increase in appetite for "comfort foods" and consequent storage of belly fat.

Americans across all age groups and geographic areas generally recognized that their stress levels are "too high" (69 percent) and that stress is not good for their health. However, a majority of respondents also reported facing significant challenges in actually practicing healthy behaviors, such as reducing stress, eating better, exercising, getting enough sleep, and losing weight. Primary obstacles to those healthy behaviors included "being too busy" (22 percent) and a "lack of motivation or willpower" (29 percent). In fact, one of the most interesting aspects of the APA survey was the clear indication that Americans know what they *should* be doing — but that they are *not* doing a good job of *achieving* their health goals. For example, if you look at the "gap" between knowing that something is important and actually doing it (achievement), we see the following pattern:

Aspects of Well-Being: Importance vs. Achievement

Behavior	Important?	Achievement?	Gap
Getting enough sleep	67%	29%	38%
Managing stress	64%	32%	32%
Eating healthy foods	58%	31%	27%
Getting enough exercise	54%	27%	27%
Having good relationships	79%	60%	19%

(Source: American Psychological Association — *Stress in America* Report [2010])

How can you close this gap? How can you break out of the negative spiral that pulls you down into burnout and turn it around toward building vigor? To answer these questions, let's look at the "central computer" that integrates the biochemical signals that, in turn, direct your behavior: your brain.

YOUR BRAIN ON STRESS

Chronic stress not only *emotionally* and *functionally* affects the brain, it can also directly *physically* affect this most important organ. Research has shown that stress not only can increase the incidence of such simple effects as "moodiness," "brain fog," or irritability, but it can also eventually progress to the development of such physical impairments as full-blown memory loss and Alzheimer's disease. Each of these conditions involves a degree of mental deterioration characterized by damage to and death of nerve cells in the brain. And it has been estimated that as many as 30 to 50 percent of adults in industrialized countries suffer from these conditions (compared to the 65 to 90 percent of adults in industrialized countries who suffer from enough chronic stress to result in *any* detrimental health condition — not just "psychological" or "brain-related" conditions).

The changes in mood that accompany periods of heightened stress also lead to reduced energy levels, feelings of fatigue, irritability, inability to concentrate, and feelings of depression — all of which are related to the same class of brain chemicals, the neurotransmitters. Most notable (and scary), perhaps, are the findings that chronic stress can lead to actual *physical* changes in the arrangement of the neurons (nerve cells) in the brain. In other words, we're talking now about stress changing both the *function* and the *structure* of your brain. No wonder your brain doesn't work the way it is supposed to!

People suffering from depression typically have disrupted biochemical balance, with imbalances in hormones, such as cortisol/

testosterone, and in brain neurotransmitters, such as dopamine, norepinephrine, and serotonin. The people who are under the highest levels of stress also tend to be the ones who succumb to periods of moderate depression. Part of the reason for this may be that during periods of heightened stress, the brain becomes accustomed to the heightened arousal signals of high cortisol levels, and when the stressor is removed (or reduced), the brain is unable to function effectively. Animal studies have shown, for example, that the brains of rats exposed to repeated stresses eventually become resistant to specific pleasure pathways; therefore, higher and higher levels of the brain's "feel-good" chemicals (dopamine, serotonin, and endorphins) were needed to induce a response. It has also been known for more than twenty years that patients given high doses of synthetic cortisol-like drugs (such as corticosteroids to treat autoimmune diseases) also tend to develop memory problems and signs of clinical depression.

The relationship between stress and brain function typically exhibits a two-phase effect, wherein short-term stress appears to actually *enhance* cognitive function, while *chronic* stress disrupts many aspects of brain neurochemistry (leaving people feeling frazzled, fatigued, and foggy). Researchers theorize that it works something like this: Acute (temporary) stress causes an increase in blood flow, oxygen, and glucose to the muscles (for activation of the fight-or-flight response) and also to the brain (sharpening mental faculties so you can "solve" the problem of escaping from the stress). Hypoglycemia (low blood sugar) can impair concentration and ability to think, so the increased supply of glucose should, at least transiently, increase brainpower. And it does; studies of people exposed to short-term stressors show that they have an enhanced memory capacity and ability for problem solving. Unfortunately, the brain-boosting effects of stress are short-lived (lasting less than thirty minutes), because then the body becomes awash in cortisol. Prolonged exposure of brain cells (neurons) to cortisol reduces their ability to take up glucose (their only fuel source) and — here's the really scary part — actually causes them to shrink in size!

NEUROPLASTICITY — CHANGING YOUR BRAIN AND BEHAVIOR

At this point, it might make perfect sense to you that the way you *think* can change the way your brain *functions* — and perhaps even that your exposure to stress and the subsequent biochemical changes in the body can further influence how your brain works. But what might sound alarming to you is that very recent scientific studies have shown that how you think and experience stress can literally change the *shape* and *structure* of your brain. Researchers have known for several decades that chronic stress can lead to accelerated *functional* impairments and eventually to *physical* degradation of brain tissue (faster breakdown and slower rebuilding). But it has only been recently that we have fully grasped the concept of "neuroplasticity" — the brain's capacity to change its *function* and its *shape* in response to experiences. The prevailing thinking in neuroscience for decades has been that the brain develops during childhood and then remains "fixed" in shape throughout adulthood. The new evidence, however, supports the exciting idea that systemic mental activity results in profound changes in the shape and structure of the brain *itself*. This means that you can literally "rewire" your brain to function better and more efficiently. You can improve the quality of the 100 billion neurons and their 100 trillion connections to improve your vigor and how you feel and perform on a daily basis.

Sports psychologists have known for decades that athletes can use "mental imagery" (basically, *thinking* about their events) to *improve* physical performance. Elite-level athletes routinely train their *bodies* for strength, speed, and agility — and the very best of the best also train their *minds* and their *emotions* for optimal performance. The average person has little understanding or appreciation for the fact that it is possible to train and to sculpt mental circuits just as biceps or buttocks can be shaped. The process is a little more complex than the simplistic "think and grow rich" platitudes that you hear from self-help gurus, but the general idea is similar. Like sand on a beach or snow on a ski slope, the brain bears the footprints or ski tracks of the decisions that you make, the experiences that you have, and the thoughts that you think. In response to the experiences and actions that you undergo, your brain strengthens the neural connections involved in these experiences and weakens those that are less frequently used. This poses important possibilities for those individuals who are troubled by depression or anxiety, making it possible to "rewire" those areas of the brain (those "pathological" connections) and establish new, better, and healthier connections that lead them away from burnout and toward vigor. Think of "problems" — such as depression, anxiety, fatigue, or burnout — as issues that involve biochemical imbalance, "faulty wiring," or a combination of both. Rebalancing either your neuronal activity or your internal biochemistry (or both) helps restore vigor as well as mood, energy, and mental focus.

Professional sports teams and international sports organizations spend millions of dollars every season to ensure their athletes are at their peak mental and physical performance levels. These teams understand that *thinking* something produces effects in the brain (and thus in the body) just as surely as *doing* something. And just as *doing* the right things in terms of diet and exercise helps the athlete excel, so does *thinking* the right things (or avoiding thinking the wrong things). Far from being "soft" sciences, the fields of "positive psychology" and sports psychology have shown over and over again in rigorous research studies that, although the brain certainly comes "hardwired" in some respects (with fear of the unknown, for example), people have an almost limitless ability to rewire their brains for change. Brains are "plastic," meaning they are malleable — changeable — and can be reeducated by specific thoughts and actions.

According to an old saying in neuroplasticity research, "Cells that fire together, wire together" — meaning that the neurons and the entire brain undergo *physical* changes in response to thoughts and experiences. This "firing/wiring together" is one reason that old habits are so difficult to break, and it explains why it takes time to establish new habits. Another reason for the "slowness" of brain changes is that neurons are slow-growing cells — much slower than liver or skin cells, which are regenerated quite rapidly, or even bone or muscle cells, which have "medium" regeneration rates. Neurons do not divide and do not "regenerate" as other body cells do. However, the human brain does possess the capacity to generate new neurons through a process called "neurogenesis," which occurs in a population of cells known as "neuronal stem cells" that can generate entirely new neurons when needed. *Most importantly, exercise stimulates this process of neurogenesis, which increases vigor. By contrast, stress hormones kill neurons and suppress neurogenesis, which reduces vigor.*

An interesting aspect of neuroplasticity is that structural brain changes seem to only occur when the mind is in a state marked by attention and focus. For example, studies of rodents have demonstrated that although *voluntary* treadmill running increases neurogenesis, *forced* running does not. Exactly *why* this difference exists is not entirely clear, but it means those who wish to change their brains or to improve their states of vigor might want to pay particular attention to the discussion of mindfulness later in this chapter. In short, you are able, in some respects, to "think your way" to certain types of change. But you also have to *want* to change for those thoughts, wishes, and desires to gain traction and result in meaningful neurogenesis. It is only through this neurogenesis of individual cells that you can make wholesale changes in brain structure and function (neuroplasticity) and establish new "tracks" that will last long enough for you to form new habits and behaviors that increase vigor.

SWITCHES AND THERMOSTATS —
ADJUSTING YOUR BRAIN CHEMISTRY

The previous chapter examines the idea that chronic stress interferes with internal biochemical balance and, further, that interference leads to imbalances that directly reduce vigor and promote burnout. However, it is possible to restore biochemical balance and, in doing so, it becomes possible to beat burnout and to reestablish a desired state of high vigor. In addition, your thoughts and experiences can alter your neural circuits and change the structure and function of your brain. This concept of neuroplasticity is also a two-way street, in that negative thoughts and actions can establish circuitry that is detrimental to your health and well-being (thus reducing vigor). On the other hand, positive thoughts and actions establish patterns of neuronal firing that promote feelings of well-being, abundant energy, and high vigor.

Because the concepts of biochemical balance and neuroplasticity can become extremely complex (and are actually not even fully understood by researchers), I often use the analogy of "switches and thermostats" to help people understand exactly what is going on at the cellular level when they are exposed to chronic stress. Think of stress as a "switch." When you're under a lot of stress, your switch is flipped "on," and when things are calm, your stress switch is in the "off" position. The switch (on or off) represents the degree of "signal" that is being transmitted to your body and to every individual cell in every tissue and organ. A constant signal from a switch that is in the "on" position for too long can overload the cell, leading to cellular dysfunction, tissue breakdown, stress-related disease, and low vigor.

Now, let's turn our attention to the "thermostat," which represents the "receptors" on the surface of cells. These receptors are the parts of the cell that transmit and interpret the signals from the switches — basically letting the cells "hear" what is going on around them. The more thermostats you have in a room of your house (or receptors on a cell), the more specifically you can detect the signal from the stress switch. Chronic stress is like having your switch in the "always on" position. When you look at the thermostats, however, you'll see that by having *more* thermostats (receptors) or having really *sensitive* thermostats that can detect very slight changes in temperature, your cells can respond quickly and very specifically to changes in the level of your stress signal. This is how your body should work when you're in good health: When you encounter stress, your switch sends the stress signal throughout the body (via nerves, hormones, neurotransmitters, cytokines, and so forth). These signals are "read" by your cellular thermostats (receptors), thus triggering actions within the cells, such as the fight-or-flight response or an increase/decrease in inflammation levels and blood sugar. Unfortunately, with chronic stress, these signals become too strong or come too frequently, so your "thermostats" begin to malfunction or shut off, and your cells no longer respond appropriately. This "insensitivity" of your "thermostats" (receptors) to the stress signals from your "switch" underlies many of the problems with biochemical balance that result in low vigor and detrimental neuroplastic changes in brain structure. Those changes cause further biochemical imbalances and reduce vigor even more in a vicious downward cycle.

TRAIN YOUR BRAIN TO BUILD VIGOR

You've just gotten a great deal of technical information about the brain, stress, and biochemistry. In this closing section of the chapter, I want to give you practical ways to apply this information to your life to change your behavior and build vigor.

Let me start by telling you about the work I've done over the years with elite-level athletes in a variety of sports — including many professional athletes and participants in the Summer and Winter Olympic Games. A common theme among these athletes and "peak-performance" enthusiasts is that the athletes standing on the podium not only are the athletes with the highest states of *physical* performance but also are the athletes with the highest states of *mental* performance and the highest states of biochemical balance and vigor (timed perfectly to coincide with their most important competitions). The athletes who miss the podium (or even miss qualifying for big events, such as the Olympic Games) are often those whose biochemistry is "unbalanced" and whose vigor slipped at the wrong time — leaving them fatigued, unfocused, injured, or sick and allowing a high-vigor athlete to surpass them. Sometimes, athletes and coaches refer to this state of high vigor as "the zone" to indicate an athlete who has momentum and who is simply "floating" out of reach of his or her competition. This "zone" is hard to describe in words (just like vigor), but when you feel it, you want to maintain it (just like vigor) — and when you lose it, you want to get it back as quickly as possible (just like vigor).

In the same way that an elite athlete must properly train body and mind to reach the highest levels of performance, you, too, must "train" yourself on a daily basis to achieve your optimal state of vigor. Over the years, I have found that two "practice sessions" are particularly effective in helping people harness and direct the power of the brain to improve personal vigor — and they are well worth a few minutes of daily practice. These two approaches are quite simple and involve practicing gratitude and mindfulness.

Let me close this chapter by offering you the following tools for incorporating gratitude and mindfulness into your life to improve the quality of your health and to build vigor.

◈ Gratitude and Mindfulness

Gratitude is the practice of focusing on what you *have* instead of what you *lack*. You may have heard the old proverb (one my grandmother used to remind me of as a child), "If you're not thankful for what you have, you're not likely to be thankful for what you'll get." One of the easiest and most effective ways to practice gratitude is to keep a "gratitude journal" in which you write down a few thoughts every week about the things for which you are grateful. You can express your gratitude in innumerable ways from past memories, present experiences, and even future hopes. These will often be "little" things, like a sunny day or a phone call from a friend — and you should write them down (or at least think about them for a few moments, like a nightly prayer) and reflect on the details of the event and the sensations that you experienced. It might sound overly simplistic, but dozens of research studies show that those who write about gratitude feel better about their lives, are significantly more optimistic, and have higher vigor.

Mindfulness is the practice of purposely focusing your attention on the present moment so you are aware and accepting, but not judgmental, of your present circumstances. When you are being mindful, you are able to savor your pleasurable experiences as they occur. You're able to derive the highest level of pleasure from each and every experience through every moment of every day. You might realize that "multitasking" is the opposite of being mindful — and you're correct. You simply cannot be mindful of anything if you're trying to pay attention to several things at the same time — for example, eating lunch while scanning e-mail and also talking on the phone means that you're not capable of deriving the pleasure you could from any one of these actions alone. People who multitask on a regular basis typically report feeling "disconnected," with lower vigor than they "should" have. But mindfulness practice can quickly restore their connection with the present and help restore their vigor. Mindfulness helps you become fully engaged in daily activities and also increases your capacity to deal with adverse events. By refocusing on the "here and now" in your daily life, mindfulness helps you worry less about the future or regret the past. You can approach mindfulness as formal meditation or less formally (as I do) when you have a moment of "downtime" (such as commuting to/from work or waiting in line). Here are a few pointers to help you focus your attention on the present:

* Focus your attention on the sensations in your body.
* Breathe in slowly and deeply through your nose, letting your chest and abdomen expand fully.
* Breathe out slowly through your mouth, letting your chest and abdomen fall as you notice the sensations of inhaling/exhaling.
* Deliberately sense and pay attention to the task at hand — move slowly and notice the sights/smells/touch/sounds of the moment.
* If your mind wanders away from the task at hand, acknowledge it and then slowly/gently refocus your attention on the present moment.

Getting back to athletes and their ability to "train" their brains to build vigor — remember that vigor is characterized by physical energy and mental energy as well as by motivation, resilience, optimism, and engagement. These are all factors that are high in a top-level athlete and are low in a poor-performing athlete. Numerous researchers in "sports psychology" have suggested that exercise training and mind training can increase positive emotions that can change brain levels of neurotransmitters (dopamine, serotonin, norepinephrine, and the natural endorphins and endocannabinoids responsible for a "runner's high"). This is yet another two-way street where the neurochemicals influence mood — and mood influences neurochemicals in either a positive or negative direction.

As stated earlier in this chapter, biochemistry affects the brain, which in turn affects behavior, and it all happens in an ongoing loop. By engaging in mindfulness and gratitude practices, you can turn this cycle away from behaviors that promote burnout and direct it toward building vigor.

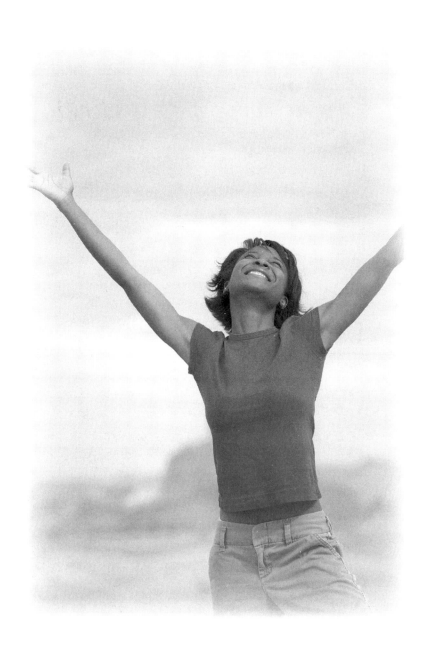

PART II *Restoring Vigor —*
The Four Pillars of Health

As you may recall from the Introduction, the Four Pillars of Health are:

1. manage oxidation
2. control inflammation
3. stabilize glucose
4. balance stress hormones

These Four Pillars offer a multipronged approach to simultaneously addressing multiple causes of biochemical imbalance. These internal processes can, in many ways, be thought of as a "Unified Theory" for promoting vigor.

By contrast, some health programs and products focus on controlling *only* inflammation, *only* oxidation, *only* blood sugar, and so forth. Although these approaches have some value, single-focus programs are automatically limited in their overall effects. Limited programs with limited focuses lead to limited benefits for you. Many of these solitary approaches offer *some* hope and *some* help. But the Four-Pillars approach enables you to balance each of the major biochemical aspects of health and vigor at the same time.

For example, scientists and doctors agree that excessive inflammation can lead to accelerated tissue damage and breakdown, so it makes a lot of sense to control inflammation to promote overall health. But, if you look deeper to find the causes of inflammation, you quickly see other factors that you can control. Because oxidation (which is caused by free radicals) leads to inflammation at the cellular level, why not also control oxidation? Great idea — but why not look even farther up the metabolic chain of events to see if you can control or modulate the causes of oxidation? Doing this shows that glycation (cellular damage caused by overexposure to certain sugars) can lead to oxidation (which can, in turn, lead to inflammation). That means you have another factor that you can address (as you do with Health Pillar 3 — stabilize glucose). Should you stop there? Of course not, because when you look even higher up the metabolic stream, you see that an imbalance in stress hormones can lead to glycation, which can lead to oxidation, which in turn leads to inflammation. Unfortunately, existing scientific or medical research doesn't go any farther "upstream" with regard to the biochemistry of cellular aging and health promotion. Balancing stress hormones is about as far "upstream" as you can go at this time — but that's still pretty good.

Obviously, each of these four aspects of your body's biochemistry is intimately intertwined and interdependent on the others. Having an imbalance in any of the individual pillars (inflammation, for example) can set off a biochemical cascade leading to imbalances in another pillar (such as oxidation). The pillars act almost like a set of dominoes — when you touch one, you set off movement and changes in all the others. The good news is that when you *restore* balance in any of the pillars, you can also get the benefit of restored balance in the rest of them, with the end result being optimal levels of health. This section of the book tells you more about these pillars and how you can reach those higher levels of health to develop vigor.

3

Health Pillar 1 —
Manage Oxidation

If you've ever noticed an apple turning brown shortly after being cut open or an old car with rust spots all over it, you've actually seen the results of a natural process called "oxidation." Within the body, oxidation takes place on the cellular level, and that is the focus of this chapter, because managing oxidative balance is the first key pillar of health for building vigor.

One simple definition of oxidation is that it describes what happens when oxygen combines with another substance. On a somewhat more technical level, oxidation refers to the loss of "at least one electron when two or more substances interact."

How are these electrons lost? They're "stolen" by highly reactive oxygen molecules called "free radicals." Many health-conscious readers are familiar with the term "antioxidant" and understand that it refers to such nutrients as vitamins C and E, among others, that help protect the body from these "free radicals."

Free radicals are highly reactive and potentially damaging, because they have an "unpaired" electron that wants to "pair" with another electron. Unfortunately, free radicals often try to "take" that needed electron from proteins and lipids in the cells, creating microscopic damage to cellular structures and leading to tissue dysfunction. Perhaps even worse than the direct damage to DNA and cellular structures is that damage in one part of the cell can set off a chain reaction of damage that can be propagated from one part of the cell to another, just as a campfire spark jumps from tree to tree in a forest and leads to a wildfire. Free radicals are not necessarily "bad" — a certain amount of cellular "damage" is actually needed for normal physiological functioning, including normal glucose transport, mitochondrial genesis, and muscle hypertrophy. However, unchecked or excessive free-radical activity is what leads to cellular damage — oxidation — and the cycle of inflammation and tissue dysfunction that follows.

Cells are typically able to protect themselves from free-radical damage through internal antioxidant enzymes produced in the body (superoxide dismutase, glutathione peroxidase, catalase) as well as through antioxidant nutrients found in the diet (vitamins C and E, thiols, flavonoids, and carotenoids — each of which can "quench" free radicals by donating their own electrons).

THE FREE RADICAL THEORY OF DISEASE

As you've just learned, when your body's own internal antioxidant defenses are overwhelmed by free radicals, damage may occur to DNA, proteins, and lipids in cell membranes (generally referred to as "lipid peroxidation"). Excessive free-radical production can come from air pollution, cigarette smoke, intense exercise, and even immune-system activity (this is because immune cells release superoxide, hydrogen peroxide, and nitric oxide as part of their "respiratory burst" to kill pathogens and clear out damaged cell material).

The most common free radicals in the body include superoxide (O_2-), hydrogen peroxide (H_2O_2), hydroxyl radical (OH-), nitric oxide (NO-), and peroxyl radical (NOO-). Superoxide, the most reactive of the free radicals, is formed in the mitochondria of the cell during the normal passage of molecular oxygen through the electron transport chain during creation of ATP (adenosine triphosphate) for cellular energy. Superoxide is inactivated by the action of the cellular antioxidant enzyme, superoxide dismutase, resulting in hydrogen peroxide. At this stage, it is still a free radical, but one with a lower potency. Hydrogen peroxide can be further converted into harmless water and oxygen by the activity of other cellular antioxidant enzymes, catalase, and glutathione peroxidase.

The free-radical theory of aging and disease promotion holds that through a gradual accumulation of microscopic damage to cell membranes, DNA, tissue structures, and enzyme systems, people begin to lose function and are predisposed to disease — not to mention a loss of vigor. In response to free-radical exposure, the body increases its production of endogenous antioxidant enzymes (such as glutathione peroxidase, catalase, and superoxide dismutase). But it has been theorized that, in some situations, it may be necessary to supplement the dietary intake of antioxidants to help prevent excessive oxidative damage to muscles, mitochondria, lungs, and other tissues — especially during or following intense exercise and exposure to pollutants, such as secondhand smoke or oxidizing radiation from sunlight.

MANAGE OXIDATION TO INCREASE VIGOR

Now that you have been introduced to the concept of oxidation and learned a little about how it contributes to cellular damage, it is time to consider what you can do to manage this process to increase your level of vigor. Remember, as long as the body is not overrun by free radicals, it can generally prevent or repair normal, day-to-day oxidative damage. The trick to fighting those free radicals, as with so many other aspects of health, is to find the right balance — specifically, the right balance of antioxidants.

When it comes to antioxidant nutrition, your best approach is to eat five to ten servings of brightly colored fruits and vegetables throughout the day. In general, brighter is better, with each color group representing a major class of antioxidants: Think orange carrots (beta-carotene), red tomatoes (lycopene), blueberries (flavonoids), and purple grapes (anthocyanins). Try to get a few servings of each color group every day, because, even though a particular "color" indicates a predominant family of antioxidant nutrients, each fruit or vegetable choice also contains hundreds of other antioxidant nutrients that work together to deliver balanced protection against free radicals.

If you have trouble consuming all the fruits and vegetables that you need, and you choose to supplement your diet to boost your antioxidant levels, then keep this in mind: *It is the overall collection of several antioxidants that's important, not any single "super" antioxidant.* Often, you'll see advertisements touting the "best" or "most powerful" antioxidant nutrient. But recent research clearly shows that supplementing with *too many* isolated or unbalanced antioxidants may be even worse for long-term health than getting *too few* antioxidants. Excessive levels of antioxidant supplementation (for example, too much isolated vitamin E or beta-carotene), can actually lead to *more* oxidation and tissue damage rather than protection from oxidation. That happens because, under certain circumstances, excessive doses of unbalanced dietary *anti*oxidants can become *pro*-oxidants. In other words, instead of fighting oxidation, the excess intake of these nutrients can actually promote it.

As stated above — and it is worth stating again, because it is a crucial point — when it comes to antioxidant supplementation, "more" is not "better," because it is the overall collection of and balance between several antioxidants that is important rather than any single "super" antioxidant. This concept of balancing supplemental antioxidants is referred to as the "Antioxidant Network." This network generally comprises five major classes of antioxidants, as shown below:

The Antioxidant Network

1. carotenoids (including beta-carotene, lycopene, and lutein)

2. vitamin E "complex" (tocopherols/tocotrienols)
3. vitamin C "complex" (ascorbic acid plus bioflavonoids)
4. thiols (e.g., sulfur-containing compounds, such as alpha-lipoic acid and cysteine)
5. bioflavonoids (vitamin-like phytonutrients, including polyphenols from citrus and berries, xanthones from mangosteen, and catechins from tea)

In theory, smaller doses of these antioxidant agents, when combined, will help combat free radicals directly. Further, they could also regenerate one another following free-radical quenching, thus delivering a more-effective and safer antioxidant regimen than with higher doses of isolated antioxidant nutrients. This combined approach to antioxidant supplementation is also logical, because certain antioxidants will work primarily against certain free radicals and in specific parts of the body (for example, vitamin E against hydroxyl radicals and within cell membranes or vitamin C against superoxide and within aqueous spaces).

Thousands of studies have clearly documented the beneficial effects of dozens of antioxidant nutrients, and thousands of nutrients and phytochemicals possess significant antioxidant activity. Increased dietary intake of antioxidant nutrients — such as vitamins C and E, such minerals as selenium, and various phytonutrients, such as extracts from grape seed, pine bark, and green tea — have all been linked to reduced rates of oxidative damage. This intake of antioxidants may also help reduce the incidence of such chronic diseases as heart disease and cancer.

But *megadose* supplementation with antioxidants can easily become a case of "too much of a good thing" and actually begin to interfere with normal cellular metabolism. This concept of antioxidant network *balance* — not too few, but also not too many — requires remembering that cells need representatives from each and every one of these categories to mount the strongest antioxidant defense. Think of it in sports terms: Even if you were the best swimmer in the world (say, Olympic gold medalist Michael Phelps), you're not going to win the Ironman triathlon without also being a strong cyclist and runner. The analogy of baseball works as well. If your team included the best homerun hitter in the world but poor pitching and fielding, then your baseball team would probably not win the World Series. The same thing holds true with your antioxidant defenses — green tea, vitamin E, or beta-carotene are all wonderful antioxidants on their own, but combining them to create a network that *performs together* in *different parts* of the body and against *different types* of free radicals is most effective.

Just as with other aspects of your health and lifestyle, if you keep the concept of "balance" in mind when it comes to your antioxidant nutrition, then your body will be healthier, stronger, and more able to respond to the demands of living, working, and "playing" at the highest level possible.

NOTE: For more detailed information on the pros, cons, safety, and dosage recommendations for specific antioxidant nutrients (and hundreds of other supplements), visit SupplementWatch at www.supplementwatch.com and Natural Medicines Comprehensive Database at www.naturaldatabase.com.

PILLAR POINTS TO REMEMBER...

Let's recap the process of oxidation, because excessive oxidation saps vigor, and managing this process is one way to strengthen this key pillar of health.

Overexposure to free radicals — and the cellular "oxidative" damage they can cause — leads to tissue dysfunction, DNA damage, reduced mitochondrial-energy production, and the ill health that you generally recognize as aging and burnout, which represents a complete loss of vigor. Too much oxidation is bad — got it?

Free radical damage can be reduced by the balanced activity of internal antioxidant enzymes and dietary antioxidant nutrients — remember, not too few *or* too many. The sum of the Antioxidant Network is more effective than its individual parts. In practical terms, this means you want to consume a variety of antioxidant nutrients every day. For example, consuming more flavonoids (found in berries, grapes, and citrus fruits) can also prevent the oxidation and loss of vitamin C and increase cellular levels of glutathione, which can switch on DNA-repair enzymes and help regulate chronic inflammation and immune function.

Unfortunately, when building vigor, you can't just manage oxidation and stop there, because the process of oxidation also impacts inflammation — most notably and directly via the activity of your immune system. The next chapter, "Health Pillar 2 — Control Inflammation," delves into this issue more deeply.

THE PILLARS IN ACTION
(VIGOR, ENERGY, AND IMMUNE FUNCTION)

Nora was a first-grade teacher who actively managed oxidation to improve her vigor. At forty-four years old, with nearly twenty years of teaching experience, Nora, like a lot of teachers, suffered from daily fatigue and a high susceptibility to catching colds. She was already taking large doses of vitamin C to try to "stimulate" her immune system, but it didn't seem to help until she added the other components of the Antioxidant Network (vitamin E, xanthones/ flavonoids, thiols, carotenoids) and beta-glucan to support immune-system function (a major source of oxidation in the body). Along with these dietary supplements, Nora also incorporated Vigor Improvement Practices, including getting eight hours of sleep on most nights and writing in her gratitude journal before bed.

Within one month, Nora's Vigor Score had improved from Low (25 points) to High (5 points). She finally had abundant energy during the day for her students and in the evenings for her family, and for the first time in many years of teaching, she used zero sick days across an entire school year.

4

Health Pillar 2 —
Control Inflammation

The word "inflammation" is derived from the Latin "*inflammare*" — meaning to "set on fire" — because an injury or infection is typically red, warm, and painful. Think of pain and inflammation as different sides of the same coin (front and back or heads and tails, whichever analogy you prefer). The point is, pain and inflammation are driven by different — but *related* — biochemical factors. The good news is that a number of natural options are safe and effective for controlling pain and inflammation — and you'll get a better idea of what some of those options are later in this chapter.

Pain and inflammation are normal body processes. Without them, you would literally not be able to survive for very long. Pain is a signal to your body that damage is occurring, and you need to stop doing whatever is causing that damage. Inflammation is a process controlled by the immune system that protects your body from invading bacteria and viruses, but this process also helps regulate heart function, blood flow, and many vital functions. Maintaining a normal balance of pain signals and inflammation is critical to good health and vigor.

When this balance becomes disrupted, you experience more inflammation and increased pain, along with less flexibility and reduced mobility. When you have too much inflammation, this process — which is supposed to be *protecting* you — actually *causes* more and more damage. For example, an *overactive* inflammatory response is known to stimulate bone breakdown (leading to osteoporosis), interfere with cartilage repair (leading to a worsening of arthritis), and accelerate muscle breakdown (leading to flareups in fibromyalgia). Inflammation is also involved in emotional balance and brain function. So when your body experiences too much inflammation, you simply don't feel happy. Instead you feel mentally exhausted and burned out — obviously, the opposite of vigor.

Your doctor may also give your *unbalanced inflammation* another kind of label — one that ends in "-itis." In medical terminology, "-itis" is used to denote inflammation. Therefore, you may have arthr*itis* (inflammation of the joint — "*arthros*" is Latin for joint), tendon*itis* (inflammation of the tendon), or fasci*itis* (inflammation of the fascia — the tough layer of connective tissue over muscles, tendons, and ligaments that can become inflamed following excessive exercise or with lower-back pain and fibromyalgia).

NORMAL INFLAMMATION
VERSUS CHRONIC INFLAMMATION

The normal process of inflammation helps dismantle and recycle older tissues that have become damaged or worn out or that simply need repair. This process is called "turnover," or "normal inflammation," and it occurs when older tissue is replaced with newer tissue. Before the age of thirty or so, this normal turnover process is perfectly balanced — for every bit of tissue that is damaged and removed, another similar (or greater) bit is put in its place. This means that, under ordinary circumstances, you're always making your tissue stronger and more resilient. After about age thirty, however, the turnover process becomes somewhat less efficient year after year. This causes a very slight loss of healthy tissue — you continue to break down and to remove some tissue, but the amount of healthy tissue added back is just a little bit less than it should be. As you age, the turnover process becomes less and less efficient, and your body's ability to heal itself from injury is reduced. This imbalance in tissue turnover and the "normal inflammation" process is the primary cause of the loss of flexibility, vigor, and the various "-itis" diseases that people tend to encounter as they get older.

With aging, these normal repair mechanisms start to dwindle, and, ironically, the very inflammatory process that has been helping "turn over" older tissue into healthy new tissue can completely *turn on you*. That leads to problems with pain, mobility, and flexibility. The same process of inflammation that naturally governs your body's repair and protection starts to accelerate tissue breakdown and impede that repair. The end result, as you may have already started to experience, is that your tissues literally begin to fall apart. Cartilage degrades, muscles lose tone, ligaments and tendons creak, bones become brittle, energy and mood falter, and vigor is sapped.

Let's keep in mind that not all inflammation is bad. As you've just learned, inflammation is part of the normal healing and turnover process for any tissue. But when you experience *too much* inflammation, things go awry. In this chapter, this state of "too much" inflammation is referred to as "chronic inflammation." With chronic inflammation, healing is suppressed, and tissue destruction is accelerated. Your body simply cannot heal itself or stop the damage when inflammation gets out of control. To illustrate this point, think about the ocean crashing against a protective seawall. The seawall represents your tissues, and the ocean is your inflammatory process. Over time, that wall will become broken and weakened by the crashing waves and will need to be repaired to return to optimal functioning. If the pace of repair fails to keep up with the pace of destruction, then the seawall fails, and the ocean comes rushing in (leading to tissue destruction and dysfunction). You need to maintain the integrity of the seawall (your tissue) by keeping up with repair and maintenance — but you can't do that if the ocean is continually crashing down on you.

A plethora of scientific and medical evidence demonstrates how to use diet, exercise, and supplementation to "calm" the ocean (to reduce damage caused by excessive inflammation) and to accelerate tissue repair (to keep that seawall intact). *It is all a question of balance.* You want to maintain a normal level of inflammation so you can then maintain a normal pace of tissue turnover and thus retain healthy tissue, flexibility, and mobility. As soon as you get too much inflammation — that is, chronic inflammation — even by a small amount, you see a little bit more tissue deterioration, leading to a little more inflammation and still more tissue breakdown. Once this vicious cycle of inflammation/damage has begun, it can be very difficult to stop — unless you have a comprehensive plan to control inflammation via multiple health practices.

CHRONIC INFLAMMATION — THE WORLD ON FIRE

It may help you to think of chronic inflammation as you would a fire in an apartment building. Let's say you live in a twenty-story apartment building, which represents your body. Then, a fire (inflammation) breaks out on the fifteenth floor, causing destruction (tissue damage) to the entire floor. But your penthouse apartment on the twentieth floor is fine. To put out the fire, you call in the firefighters (immune cells), which may cause a bit more damage by tearing down some walls and spraying water (cytokines, a substance secreted by immune system cells), all in an effort to solve the bigger problem of putting out the fire. Let's now say that the fifteenth floor is a complete loss, while other floors suffer some repairable damage (water damage on the fourteenth floor and smoke damage on the sixteenth floor). The repair process begins on all three floors, with carpenters, painters, and other "builders" brought in to repair the damage. On floors fourteen and sixteen, where the damage is less severe, the repair process might be complete within a few weeks, but on the fifteenth floor, where the fire was concentrated and the damage was most severe, the repair process may take a year.

Your body also has an entire team of "builder" cells in each and every tissue. In cartilage these "builders" are called chondrocytes, in bone they are called osteoblasts, in muscles they are myocytes, in skin and some other tissues they are fibroblasts — the list goes on and on. In your own tissues, you can have the equivalent of a raging fire and a firefighting team (tissue damage and inflammation). But if you're not able to shut off this process — that is, if your level of inflammation is thrown off by something — then your body is in a continual state of destruction and pain. You'll never be able to get to the rebuilding and repair stages unless you can shut off this process of chronic inflammation.

THE BIOCHEMISTRY OF INFLAMMATION

Much of the body's inflammatory response is regulated by two enzymes: cyclooxygenase ("COX" for short) and lipoxygenase (abbreviated as "LO"). The COX enzyme can be further divided into COX-1 and COX-2. Often, COX-1 is referred to as being the "good" form, because it protects the stomach and kidneys. COX-2, however, is labeled the "bad" form of the enzyme, because it is responsible for creating inflammatory chemicals called prostaglandins from a dietary and cellular fat called arachidonic acid. Two other related LO (lipoxygenase) enzymes are also involved in the inflammation process: "5-LO" and "12-LO." Both work a little differently to convert arachidonic acid into highly inflammatory compounds known as thromboxanes and eicosanoids. It makes a lot of sense, therefore, to control COXs and LOs at the same time.

Dozens of natural options allow you to control COX-2 *and* 5-LO *and* 12-LO, while leaving COX-1 alone to continue protecting your gut — but *zero* drugs can do all this. Why? Mostly, because a multinational drug company can't make a billion dollars a year in profits by selling natural extracts of leaves or roots. Instead, it can create its own "better" synthetic version of nature, patent it, and sell it at high profits with the blessing of the Food and Drug Administration (FDA). Natural products, on the other hand, can work just as well (and in some cases better) as many synthetic drugs, can work in ways that the drugs can't, and can deliver benefits without the side effects that are all too common with the growing array of drugs entering the market each year.

In the early 1990s, the drug companies figured that if they could create a molecule that was capable of stopping only the COX-2 enzyme while leaving COX-1 alone, then they might be able to control pain and inflammation without the nasty side effects associated with such drugs as ibuprofen (Advil), naproxen (Aleve), and aspirin. Each of these drugs can get rid of your headache, but they can also destroy your stomach lining and your kidneys, because they all interfere with COX-1 *and* COX-2. The idea of creating a *selective* COX-2 inhibitor was a good one ("on paper," as they say) — except for the fact that even after drug companies learned these drugs were causing heart attacks and strokes, they insisted on continuing to sell them at huge profits. You can learn more about this issue in Appendix B.

As drug companies will often do, they looked first to nature to see whether any plants, herbs, or other natural products contained any clues to the inhibition of the COX enzyme. Lo and behold! They found hundreds of plants and herbs with powerful anti-inflammatory and pain-controlling effects (such as ginger, turmeric, and mangosteen) — some via the COX enzymes, some via the 5-LO enzyme, and others through completely novel biochemical mechanisms. Also, as drug companies will *always* do, they took this knowledge and turned their backs on nature, arrogantly believing that they could "do better" by synthetically creating a new-to-the-world molecule that more powerfully interfered with the inflammatory enzymes. The result was Celebrex, which inhibits

COX-2 about four hundred times more powerfully than it does COX-1; and Vioxx, which inhibits COX-2 about one thousand times more powerfully than COX-1 (and which has subsequently been pulled off the market). These drugs are marvels of synthetic chemical engineering to be sure, but they are also prime examples of science run amok in the pursuit of profits. You've probably heard your mother say something like, "You'd cut off your own nose to spite your face," when you were being unreasonable as a child. Well, the "COX-2" class of drugs was exactly the same scenario, with drug companies encouraging consumers to gulp drugs that controlled inflamed and achy knees but destroyed hearts and blood vessels. It is a sad state of affairs when average Americans are being told that they only have two choices for controlling inflammation and pain: First, take the older painkillers (NSAIDs, which are non-steroidal anti-inflammatory drugs) that temporarily relieve inflammation and pain but also wreck their stomachs; or secondly, take the newer painkillers (COX-2 inhibitors) that temporarily relieve pain but wreck their hearts. Better options do exist. (And you'll learn about a few of those options at the end of this chapter in the section titled "Control Inflammation — Naturally — For More Vigor.")

HOW NORMAL INFLAMMATION BECOMES CHRONIC

When a tissue is damaged — whether from infection, trauma, or unbalanced turnover — it releases signaling chemicals called "cytokines." These cytokines are like flare guns, sending up a call for help that signals surrounding cells to jump into action to stop (wall off) and repair the damage. The cytokines also call immune-system cells (white blood cells) into the area to help clean up the damaged tissue. You have no doubt experienced the blood rush that leads to the recognizable redness, warmth, and swelling common to many injuries. As the white blood cells rush in to the damaged area, they release more and more of their own inflammatory chemicals. This blast of inflammation is intended to cause even more tissue destruction as a way to either kill bacteria and viruses or to take away damaged tissue and set the stage for repair efforts to begin. As you can imagine, this part of the inflammatory process is supposed to be short term. If it were to continue without shutting down, you'd simply destroy your own tissue without ever rebuilding healthy tissue in its place. Unfortunately, this "never-shut-down" scenario precisely describes the chronic inflammation and constant state of tissue destruction with which millions of Americans live their lives every day.

A number of mechanisms are in place to shut down the process of inflammation, including the naturally short half-life of cytokines and other inflammatory molecules and the production of anti-inflammatory cytokines (with such names as TGF-beta and IL-10). Unfortunately, immune-system cells can remain in a state of chronic inflammation if the "cell-damage" signals keep coming to them as a result of free-radical damage (as discussed in Chapter 3) and from cortisol-induced tissue breakdown (covered in Chapter 6); or if signals to "shut down" the inflammatory process are not "heard" by target cells (as in the case of cells damaged by problems with glucose [blood-sugar] levels, a subject covered in the next chapter).

Unfortunately, chronic inflammation is not confined to the tissue in which it starts. Cytokines — such as those labeled IL-6, IL-8, and TNF-alpha — are able to leave the original site of inflammation. They can then travel in the blood to spread inflammatory signals through the blood vessels and into every tissue in the body (leading to metabolic diseases, such as obesity, diabetes, and depression, and to structural/damage diseases, such as Alzheimer's, Parkinson's, and arthritis). Because most of the cytokine molecules are produced by immune-system cells (specifically by macrophages, neutrophils, and NK cells of the innate immune system), numerous drug companies attempt to control chronic inflammation by suppressing immune function. The problem, of course, is that wholesale suppression of immune function also limits your body's ability to protect you from actual pathogens — so you're "protected" from chronic inflammation, but you may become more susceptible to infections and certain cancers. Not a great trade-off!

CHRONIC INFLAMMATION
AND CHRONIC DISEASES

Chronic inflammation is not only a problem that affects the way you feel on a daily basis or the level of vigor you experience. It also contributes to the development of serious health conditions, including four that we will briefly discuss in this section: heart disease, cancer, obesity, and diabetes.

◈ Heart Disease

Researchers probably know the most about the adverse effects of chronic inflammation when it comes to heart disease. Until about ten years ago, most cardiologists and other health experts believed that heart disease was a simple "plumbing" problem, with too much cholesterol being the culprit that clogged up blood vessels and led to heart attacks. Unfortunately, the cause of heart attacks was later determined to be a little more complicated when population studies showed that at least half of all heart attacks occurred in people with perfectly normal cholesterol levels. What scientists know now is that oxidative damage (by free radicals) is what allows cholesterol to become "sticky" in the first place and to start plugging blood-vessel linings with plaque deposits. Chronic inflammation, therefore, seems to be the "trigger" that causes those deposits to rupture and create a blockage in the heart, leading to a heart attack. The degree of chronic inflammation throughout the body can be measured by blood levels of a protein called

"C-reactive protein" (CRP). CRP is produced in the liver, with levels rising in direct proportion to inflammatory signals in the body. During times of active infection (acute inflammation), CRP levels may rise by a factor of one thousand to fifty thousand in response to the increased production of cytokines, such as IL-6, from macrophages. A CRP value of 3.0 mg/L is associated with a tripling of heart-attack risk, while people with very low CRP levels (below 0.5 mg/L) rarely have any sign of inflammatory heart disease. You may have to push for it, but you can have your CRP levels tested the next time you're in the doctor's office.

◈ Cancer

For more than one hundred years, researchers have known that cancerous tumors tend to arise and cluster at sites of chronic inflammation. Stated another way, sites of chronic inflammation seem to attract and promote the growth of cancer. Part of this effect might have to do with the fact that sites with more inflammation will also have more oxidative free-radical damage — so DNA damage and subsequent "mistakes" during repair may result in more mutations and a higher chance for cancer development. Another factor may be that a higher concentration of inflammatory cytokines attracts a greater number of immune cells, which "think" they're being called to the site of an infection and thus create even more damage as they try to "kill" a nonexistent pathogen. So here is evidence of the ultimate conundrum: Your immune cells, which normally protect you against cancer, may actually be co-opted by excessive inflammatory signals into stimulating further cancer growth.

◈ Obesity and Diabetes

Obesity is defined as an excess of adipose (fat) tissue, with adipose tissue producing a range of inflammatory cytokines (adipokines, adiponectin, leptin, resistin, TNF-alpha, IL-6, IL-1, and many others). Adiponectin and leptin are the most abundant adipokines and are considered key signaling compounds in regulating inflammation within fat cells and throughout the body. Adiponectin levels are markedly decreased in obesity, diabetes, and heart disease and are thought to contribute direct anti-inflammatory effects. Leptin, on the other hand, is considered a highly proinflammatory and proatherogenic cytokine that is associated with elevated body fat levels and reduced insulin sensitivity. The ratio between adiponectin and leptin has been proposed by some researchers as a useful index of heart-disease risk in patients with obesity and diabetes. Leptin acts directly on the hypothalamus region of the brain to regulate food intake and energy expenditure. Leptin helps the body tell the brain that the body is satiated and that enough fat is stored. The amount of leptin produced is proportional to the amount of body fat stored, so when you lose body fat, your leptin levels fall and your hunger increases to drive you to eat to "replace" the lost fat. On the other hand, adiponectin increases fat oxidation and improves the activity of insulin to regulate blood-sugar levels. Through cytokines/adipokines, fat tissue can be directly influenced by the overall inflammatory state of the body, but through the action of cytokines/adipokines on the brain, fat tissue can also influence inflammation throughout the entire body. Aside from the adipokine signaling mentioned above, another important source of chronic inflammation associated with abdominal obesity is the constant activation of the innate immune system. As they grow, changes in cell-surface proteins on adipose tissue can allow swollen abdominal fat cells to resemble bacterial cells or tumor cells in certain ways. This effect attracts cells from the innate immune system (macrophages, neutrophils, and NK cells), which attempt to destroy the "tumor" (your own fat cells) with their normal bursts of free radicals and cytokines. Unfortunately, rather than killing off your fat (if only it were that simple!), this immune system attack merely damages your fat cells, which sets off the expected normal cycle of injury/inflammation/repair that any of your body cells would undergo. The really bad news is that the end result is yet a higher level of inflammation and oxidation — and a growth of fat stores through a variety of metabolic signals.

CONTROL INFLAMMATION — NATURALLY — FOR MORE VIGOR

If the inflammation process is a multifaceted chain reaction of biochemical events, then shouldn't your approach to controlling inflammation also be multifaceted? Of course it should! This is one of the many ways in which synthetic single-action pharmaceutical drugs fail miserably. Drugs are a single molecule — a single chemical entity — that work on *one* biochemical mechanism, albeit it in a very powerful way — sometimes too powerfully, leading to serious side effects. If the recent history of medicine has demonstrated anything, it is that these single-action, modern pharmaceutical drugs, these synthetic silver bullets previously unknown in nature, can have serious adverse consequences.

Among adults, nearly 10 percent of those who use NSAIDs, such as ibuprofen, will require hospitalization due to serious gastrointestinal toxicity (such as ulcers and stomach bleeding). In a 1998 study published in the *American Journal of Medicine,* researchers reported that more than 107,000 people are admitted each year to hospitals — and another 17,000 *die* each year — as a direct result of complications due to the use of NSAIDs. This is a problem.

Popping a pill, such as an aspirin, ibuprofen, or one of the newer prescription drugs, to control your pain is certainly not the answer. Although these drugs may be able to offer a short-term reduction in sensations of pain, they do *nothing* to address the root of the problem, which is to get the inflammation process into balance. In fact, by inhibiting the COX-2 enzyme and related inflammatory pathways, such as prostaglandin production, in such a strong way, these drugs can actually *reduce* tissue repair (especially for joint cartilage) and lead to severe damage in other tissues, such as kidneys, liver, heart, and the entire gastrointestinal system (potentially leading to gastric ulcers, stomach bleeding, and even death).

As discussed earlier in the section entitled, "The Biochemistry of Inflammation," the term "COX-2 inhibitor" generally refers to synthetic pharmaceutical drugs that interfere with the key enzyme involved with increasing inflammation and pain in the body. And, as you may recall, those drugs include Vioxx and Celebrex (the first has been forced off the market for causing heart attacks, and the second is still under investigation for the same heart risks). What you may not know, however, is that thousands of years ago, ancient herbal practitioners were prescribing all-natural, herbal COX-2 inhibitors for controlling pain and inflammation. What these traditional healers did not realize at the time, but what we know now thanks to advances in nutritional biochemistry, is that these natural anti-inflammatory nutrients were effective at controlling inflammation in *many ways, simultaneously.* This balanced approach is associated not only with a greater degree of overall effectiveness but also with a restoration of normal tissue function and fewer side effects. As is so often the case, however, the drug industry has tried to synthetically copy the extraordinary healing properties and powers of natural medicine — only to cause even more suffering, injury, and death. Fortunately, those herbs and natural products cannot be "owned" by the drug companies, keeping them widely available to anyone who wants to enjoy the safe and effective benefits of controlling pain and inflammation naturally.

When it comes to selecting a natural option for inflammatory balance and pain relief ,the obvious dilemma is that you want something that is safe, natural, fast-acting, and long-lasting. It is a tall order to get all four "wants" into a single item — but a growing number of products offer a suitable range of options (mostly by combining the most effective ingredients into a single, multifaceted product solution).

Now that I've presented the idea that herbs and natural products can combat inflammation and pain, you may now be wondering what, exactly, you need to ingest to address these health issues. Let me stop you right there for a moment. To obtain the real benefits from natural products and traditional healing wisdom, you have to break out of the mind-set that tells you taking one pill or one drug will cure your ills with a "quick fix." That mind-set is pervasive in modern society, and countless ads and commercials constantly reinforce it. So before considering specific natural strategies for controlling inflammation, the first thing you need to do is to be willing to change the mind-set that says you can take a pill and forget the problem. You may also need to change your lifestyle and recognize the importance of being an active participant in developing your health and wellness, not a passive recipient of a prescription from a physician. Many of you are no doubt aware of the benefits of changing your mind-set and lifestyle to embrace a view of health that is more comprehensive and multifaceted than the typical Western medical approach. Nevertheless, it bears repeating, because even people who appreciate traditional medicine can fall back into thinking that one "superfood" or one "special" herb will solve a health problem as quickly and efficiently as a pill from the pharmacist.

Having said all that, here are a few specific, natural options that you can pursue to control inflammation and pain:

❖ *Exercise* — Numerous studies confirm that moderate exercise reduces inflammation as well as the production of C-reactive protein, which plays a role in heart disease. One study from researchers at the Emory University School of Medicine in Atlanta that was published in the *Archives of Internal Medicine* (2002) found that the more frequently you exercise, the lower your overall level of inflammation. The study looked at nearly four thousand U.S. adults ages forty and older and found that exercising approximately

five times per week was associated with almost a 40 percent reduction in overall inflammation. (See Chapter 9 for
more details on exercise.)

❧ *Sleep* — Sleep is crucial to your health and vigor in countless ways, including helping corral chronic inflammation.
In one study published in the *Archives of Internal Medicine*
(2006), researchers from the UCLA School of Medicine
found that even a single night of disrupted sleep increases
levels of inflammation throughout the body by two to
three times compared to a normal night's sleep. You'll learn
more about getting better sleep in Chapter 7.

❧ *Herbs and Supplements* — As noted earlier in this chapter,
ginger, turmeric, and mangosteen are effective dietary
supplements for reducing inflammation naturally. Many
other herbs and dietary supplements also help control inflammation. For instance, the sap or resin of the boswellia
plant has long been used in traditional Indian medicine to
treat arthritis and other inflammatory conditions. Chapter
10 includes much more information on using supplements
to address inflammation, as well as the other biochemical
processes outlined in the Four Pillars of Health.

If you are one of the twenty-five million Americans living with
chronic low-back pain and the almost forty million suffering from
arthritis, getting rid of that pain is obviously an important consideration. Natural options found in dietary supplements and other
approaches may not offer a "quick fix," and they should be viewed
not only as simple pain relievers but also as agents to enhance the
body's healing response and restore biochemical balance to the
entire inflammatory process. Most OTC (over-the-counter) an-
algesics (painkillers) and nonsteroidal anti-inflammatory drugs
(NSAIDs) are safe and effective for *short-term* usage (two to three
days at a time). NSAIDs do a great job of beating back the pound-
ing from that headache, but they don't do a thing to help promote

healing of your aching knee. In fact, in some important ways, these drugs may actually *inhibit* tissue healing, especially in the case of cartilage repair. There is also little doubt that NSAID therapy can lead to gastroduodenal ulcers, primarily due to their inhibition of prostaglandin production in the mucosal lining of the gastrointestinal tract (no mucus = no protection of stomach/intestinal lining = you digest yourself).

Coming chapters discuss more natural options for controlling inflammation and strengthening the other Pillars of Health to improve mobility and flexibility and actually rebuild damaged tissues for long-term well-being. The next chapter explores the effects that inflammatory cytokines (produced in many cells of the body, including immune cells, liver cells, and fat cells) have directly and indirectly on insulin function and blood-sugar control and how these effects, when unbalanced, drive people toward diabetes and further inflammation.

PILLAR POINTS TO REMEMBER...

As indicated in Chapter 3, the biochemical processes of oxidation and inflammation are inextricably linked — they go hand-in-hand through common immune system pathways. The immune system responds to and creates oxidative "free radicals" and responds to and creates inflammatory cytokines. (In case you've forgotten, cytokines are a class of hormonelike signaling proteins that play a role in the immune response and inflammatory levels throughout the body.)

"Normal" inflammation exists to protect us from invading pathogens (viruses, bacteria, and even uncontrolled cell growth that could lead to cancerous tumors). Sometimes, however, the walling-off and destroying process of the immune system's inflammatory response doesn't shut off the way it is supposed to. Immune-system cells, such as macrophages (which fight bacteria), neutrophils (which fight viruses), and natural killer cells (which fight tumors), respond to free radicals as if they were toxins. A small amount of free radical signaling is a "good thing" for immune cells, keeping them vigilant to defend us against "real" pathogens. However, when free radical exposure becomes excessive, immune cells release a wide array of proinflammatory cytokines, such as interleukins (IL-1, IL-6, TNF-alpha), to "wall off" tissues from further free radical damage. And that can lead to chronic inflammation as well as a cascade of diseases, including heart disease, obesity, diabetes, Alzheimer's, and certain cancers. Unfortunately, the Western lifestyle is a perfect recipe for increasing chronic inflammation, with its high intake of sugar, refined carbohydrates, and saturated fats. That diet, combined with low levels of fiber, infrequent exercise, and sleep deprivation, make it more likely that inflammation becomes too high — and stays that way.

To sum up: The walling-off aspect of the inflammatory process is an ideal response to keep viruses or bacteria from moving into other parts of your body, but free radical–generated inflammation encourages immune cells to fight "yourself" in a vicious cycle of oxidation/inflammation, which ends up creating more problems and eventually leading to a lower state of vigor.

THE PILLARS IN ACTION
(CRP, LOW-BACK PAIN, AND DEPRESSION)

Ralph was a successful real estate executive who controlled inflammation to alleviate his depression, rid himself of low-back pain, and reduce his CRP levels. If you looked up the definition of the words "busy" and "driven" in the dictionary, you would see a picture of Ralph staring back at you. As a recipient of his agency's "top-seller" award for ten years running, Ralph had no interest in "slowing down" — he loved the fast-paced world of real estate, and his business had been thriving even with the tough economy. Unfortunately, the chronic stress of being "on" 24/7 for work was starting to affect Ralph's personal and family life. Despite his financial success, Ralph never really felt "good" — he had trouble enjoying happy occasions in his nonwork life, and on more days than not, his lower back was tight and painful. The real eye-opener for Ralph was his annual executive physical exam, during which his doctor told him that his high level of inflammation (CRP) made him a "heart attack waiting to happen" and wrote him prescriptions for an antidepressant (for his low mood) and a painkiller (for his back pain).

Through a combination of Vigor Improvement Practices, including a three-times weekly Interval Walking program (less than thirty minutes per session) and daily consumption of mangosteen juice, Ralph saw his CRP levels drop from extremely high (11 mg) to very low (almost undetectable, at 0.3 mg). As a result of controlling his inflammation, Ralph was able to avoid having to start the prescription antidepressant and painkiller that his doctor had prescribed.

Ralph is still the top producer in his real estate firm, but he also feels great again, experiencing less pain, better moods, and prospects for an overall healthier future.

5

Health Pillar 3 —
Stabilize Glucose

There are many reasons to keep a tight control of glucose levels. Glucose, which you may often hear called "blood sugar," is the preferred source of energy for the brain, and glucose helps you fully metabolize calories from fat. Blood-sugar levels that drop too low may stimulate hunger and cravings, while glucose levels that rise too high will slow your ability to burn fat.

A key intermediary in the interrelationships between blood glucose, oxidation, inflammation, and stress hormones (covered in the next chapter) is the hormone insulin. Most people associate insulin problems with diabetes because of its primary role in regulating blood-sugar levels, but insulin has many additional functions in the body. Not only does insulin regulate blood-sugar levels within an extremely narrow range, but it is also responsible for getting fat stored in the fat cells (adipose tissue), getting sugar stored in the liver and muscle cells (as glycogen), and getting amino acids directed toward protein synthesis (to build muscle). Due to these varied actions, insulin is sometimes thought of as a "storage hormone," because it helps the body put all these sources of energy away in their respective "storage depots" for use later.

Because insulin stimulates fat synthesis and promotes fat storage, there is a widespread misbelief that insulin circulating in the body "induces" weight gain. This misconception has led to a variety of diets that promote the idea that weight loss can be achieved by avoiding certain foods, such as carbohydrates, that stimulate insulin secretion. Unfortunately, this simplistic view of energy metabolism is only partly correct. Proponents of these diets fail to distinguish between a *normal* insulin response to meals (in which temporarily elevated blood levels of insulin quickly return to normal levels after meals) and an *abnormal* insulin response (in which insulin levels stay elevated for prolonged periods following meals). When you eat appropriately (covered in Part III), your levels of insulin and leptin will rise appropriately following meals, providing you with appetite-controlling benefits. But they will also fall appropriately, keeping oxidation, inflammation, and other biochemical processes from getting out of control.

The abnormal insulin metabolism described above — known as insulin resistance — leads to a reduction in the body's cellular response to insulin. That reaction, in turn, interferes with regulation of blood sugar, increases appetite, and blocks the body's ability to burn fat due primarily to direct "blocking" of insulin function by cortisol, as well as indirect interference with insulin activity by oxidative free radicals and inflammatory cytokines. When insulin resistance is combined with a poor diet (high in fat and/or refined carbohydrates), the result is the metabolic condition known as Syndrome X, a disorder that can have an impact on virtually every disease process in the body.

SUGARS + PROTEINS = GLYCATION

Glycation is a process by which a sugar molecule (typically glucose or fructose) becomes bonded to a protein or lipid. Most often, glycation occurs in the body when glucose or fructose in the blood remains too high for too long and becomes bonded to cell-surface proteins. A related biochemical process called glycosylation is a very precise enzyme-controlled bonding of specific sugars to specific proteins at defined cellular sites (to help control metabolism). But compared to this precise process, glycation is actually a haphazard process that randomly adds sugars to proteins, impairing normal function and interfering with healthy cell-to-cell communication. A glycated protein — referred to as an "AGE" (advanced glycation end product) — can be highly reactive and set off a chain reaction of oxidative and inflammatory damage in whatever tissues they occur. AGEs also tend to be "cleared" from the body very slowly, so they have the potential to stimulate these chain reactions for prolonged periods of time.

Some of the main dietary offenders that lead to AGE accumulation and upset biochemical balance are high-sugar foods (such as soda, ice cream, donuts, cookies, or sugary breakfast cereals) and other foods that quickly convert to sugar or glucose in the bloodstream (like highly processed grains, such as white bread, rolls, or instant rice). Sugar can be toxic to many tissues by permanently attaching to proteins through the glycation process. Wherever sugar attaches, it triggers cellular microdamage that creates inflammation. The inflammation, in turn, produces enzymes that break down protein, thus resulting in damage to surrounding tissues. To make matters worse, glycation also leads to cross-linking of proteins, changing healthy tissues from soft, supple, and flexible to stiff, brittle, and painful. These stiffened sugar-protein bonds form in every type of tissue, including joint cartilage, muscle tendons, brain neurons, blood vessels, skin, and even immune-system cells, which is why scientists are finding links between glycation and the chronic diseases of "aging," such as cardiovascular disease, Alzheimer's disease, and arthritis.

We know from Chapter 4 that inflammation in any tissue can be caused by excessive exposure to free radicals and can lead to accelerated "aging" and generalized tissue breakdown. AGEs demonstrate a "direct" problem with cell-to-cell signaling that is compromised by sugar-coated proteins. "Indirect" damage is also caused by an AGE-stimulated increase in oxidation and inflammation.

Stress hormones, which we'll discuss in the next chapter, stimulate the creation of AGEs through an increase in blood-sugar levels.

People with diabetes are obviously at high risk for developing AGEs in a wide range of tissues because of their problems regulating blood-sugar levels. The extreme development of AGEs in diabetics is a key reason for their high rates of oxidative and inflammatory diseases, including nephropathy (kidney damage) and circulatory problems (due to blood-vessel damage).

GLYCATION AND THE GLYCEMIC INDEX

Lab researchers have assigned many foods with a rating known as the glycemic index (GI), which refers to the degree by which the food increases blood-sugar levels. For example, white bread has a GI of 69 and grapefruit has a GI of 26. Not everyone agrees on the GI of every food (more on that issue below). A food with a high GI will rapidly increase blood-sugar levels, while a food with a low GI will have a less-pronounced effect on blood-sugar levels. The glycemic index has doubtless helped nutrition researchers gain a greater understanding of the metabolic and health properties associated with many foods. For example, several good studies show that long-term consumption of a diet with a high glycemic load (GL, which is an index of GI and total carbohydrate content of the diet) is a significant predictor of systemic inflammation and eventual weight gain, as well as a significant risk factor for diabetes and cardiovascular disease. Unfortunately, the GI and the GL represent only portions of a very complicated metabolic story. To understand this "story," you might think of the GI and GL as representing a "glycation potential" that must be manifested via changes in oxidative balance and inflammatory balance.

Perhaps the biggest "problem" with the GI and the GL is that they are calculated for isolated foods. Nobody is (or should be) sitting down to a meal composed solely of white bread, puffed rice, or plain macaroni. These are all foods with high GIs and are therefore "banned" by some popular diets. From a purely practical point of view, even trying to determine the GI or GL value of a particular food is nearly impossible outside of a metabolic lab. For example, something as simple and apparently straightforward as a bowl of rice shows a huge range of measured GI values, which may be due to the different varieties of rice that are available (long grain versus short grain), their fiber content (white versus brown), and even the cooking method used to prepare the rice (boiling versus steaming versus frying). Another example is carrots. Published GI values place carrots into either a "high" GI category of 92 or a "low" GI category of 32. In addition, the GI and GL values of particular foods are significantly affected by factors that have nothing to do with the actual food, such as cooking methods (longer cooking tends to increase the GI of pasta, rice, and other foods), processing levels (smaller particle sizes tend to increase the GI of flours and other grains), and the levels of fiber, fat, and protein contained in the overall meal (higher levels of each of these components tend to reduce the GI).

Many other factors can significantly influence the GI or GL of a particular food, including the following:

- the ripeness of fruit (riper = a higher GI, due to a higher sugar content)
- the physical form of the food (for example, applesauce has a 25 percent higher GI than a whole apple)
- the proportion of different carbohydrate types in a single food (for example, rice and potatoes can have different levels of amylose, a slowly digested carbohydrate, versus amylopectin, a rapidly digested carbohydrate)
- the shape of the food (for instance, different forms of pasta can range from a GI value of 68 for macaroni to 45 for spaghetti; even linguine has a GI of 68 for thick noodles but scores a GI of 87 for thin noodles)

❧ processing methods (foods that are "more" processed tend to increase blood-sugar levels faster than those that are "less" processed, but it is exceedingly difficult to know the exact processes of grinding, rolling, and pressing that a product like muffin mix undergoes before it arrives on grocer's shelves)

❧ preparation methods (for example, the amount of heat and water used in cooking, the time of cooking, and even the size into which the food particles are chopped prior to cooking)

The problems with the GI have led many dieticians and nutritionists to simplify their recommendations by educating their clients to eat "complex" carbohydrates (starches) instead of "simple" ones (sugars) to help control blood-sugar levels. But this approach does not necessarily ensure consumption of the right foods. For example, white bread, mashed potatoes, and chocolate cake would be a poor example of a meal consisting of "complex" carbohydrates. In general terms, refined-grain products ("complex" or not) and potatoes tend to rapidly increase blood-sugar levels, unless they are combined with appropriate amounts of protein, fat, and fiber. Nuts, beans, legumes, and minimally processed grains (which may sometimes be labeled as "whole," even though they have actually been processed) tend to have only a moderate effect on blood-sugar levels. Most fruits and vegetables have a small effect on blood-sugar levels, but even these foods still need to be combined with appropriate metabolic regulators in the form of added protein/fat for optimal glucose control.

THE METABOLIC MEMORY

One of the biggest problems with the glycated proteins called AGEs, as indicated above, is that they persist in tissues for a long time after their initial creation. This allows AGE-damaged cells and tissues to continue causing damage to surrounding tissues — even long after you take steps to stabilize glucose. This effect is sometimes referred to as "metabolic memory," because it appears as if the individual tissues that have been influenced by AGEs will "remember" the damaging effects of elevated glucose and continue to send oxidative and inflammatory signals to surrounding tissues and throughout the body. Studies have shown that the longer that glucose levels remain uncontrolled (elevated), the more AGEs are created — and the longer that oxidative and inflammatory signals will persist even after glucose levels are lowered. Furthermore, the faster that glucose levels are returned to normal levels, the faster those damaging oxidative/inflammatory signals dissipate as well. Combining antioxidant/anti-inflammatory agents with glucose-lowering interventions has been shown to almost completely interrupt AGE-related tissue dysfunction (particularly in endothelial tissues, such as blood vessels). Glucose-lowering interventions can range from reducing your dietary intake of highly refined carbohydrates, such as white bread, to combining whole-grain carbohydrates with healthy fats and fiber to using specific glucose-control dietary supplements.

TO IMPROVE VIGOR — STABILIZE GLUCOSE

There are numerous ways to stabilize glucose and reduce your development of AGEs — some of which might seem quite obvious, as you'll see in the short list below. You'll also learn more about all of these recommendations in Part III, which details Vigor Improvement Practices.

Tips for Stabilizing Glucose

- Consume fewer high-sugar foods (soda, baked goods, refined carbs).
- Consume more low-sugar foods (vegetables, lean meats, healthy fats).

❧ Consume fewer fried foods (high-temperature cooking creates AGEs in the foods).

❧ Maintain healthy blood-sugar levels (80–100mg/dL) by:

- getting regular (intense) exercise
- getting eight hours of sleep each night
- incorporating stress-reduction practices into your daily life
- supplementing with specific glucose-controlling dietary supplements

PILLAR POINTS TO REMEMBER...

The next chapter explores the links between stress-hormone exposure and the other Pillars of Health; however, because cortisol (one of the primary stress hormones) has direct and indirect effects on glucose levels, it makes sense to outline a few of those effects in this chapter. Cortisol exposure stimulates a rapid increase in blood-glucose levels via several mechanisms, including stimulating the release of glucose stored in the liver, interfering with insulin's action to stimulate cells to absorb glucose from the blood, and stimulating the appetite with specific cravings for sweets.

Adding to the connection between cortisol and insulin resistance are a series of studies showing that inadequate sleep causes insulin resistance. This is particularly interesting because of the well-known link between sleep deprivation and elevated cortisol levels. Sleep researchers from the University of Chicago and several other universities have shown that inadequate sleep leads to a cascade of events, starting with increased cortisol levels, which induces insulin resistance, leading to higher blood-sugar (glucose) levels, causing increased measures of oxidative and inflammatory damage, stimulating appetite, and eventually leading to abdominal fat gain. The research team compared "normal" sleepers (averaging eight hours of sleep per night) to "short" sleepers (averaging six hours or less of sleep per night). They found that the "short" sleepers secreted 50 percent more cortisol and insulin and were 40 percent less sensitive to the effects of insulin than the "normal" sleepers. The researchers also suggested that sleep deprivation plays a significant role in the current epidemic of obesity and type 2 diabetes. These research results are a concern for anyone who wants to balance their blood-sugar levels — especially in light of statistics from the National Sleep Foundation, which show a steady decline in the number of hours that Americans sleep each night. In 1910 the average American slept about nine hours per night, whereas today people average only about seven hours of sleep per night — and many get far less than that — much to the detriment of vigor.

THE PILLARS IN ACTION
(ACNE, BELLY FAT, AND MENTAL FOCUS)

Tricia was a nurse and single mother of two teenage girls who stabilized glucose to enhance her mental function and reduce her belly fat. As a nurse, Tricia worked long, stressful hours and often pulled double shifts to earn extra money to support her daughters. As a single mom, Tricia had very little "downtime," and she especially had trouble finding the time to prepare healthy meals. As a result, she and her daughters frequently ate fast food and other prepared packaged foods (low in fiber and high in refined carbohydrates). Tricia knew that she and her daughters should be eating better and that doing so could also help her lose some of the belly fat that she had gained over the last few years, but all the "diets" she read about had complicated recipes or long lists of "banned" foods — neither of which would work in a household with two picky teenagers.

By incorporating a few simple Vigor Improvement Practices related to healthy nutrition choices, Tricia was able to stabilize glucose for herself and her daughters. As a family, Tricia and her daughters agreed to give up soda (full-sugar and artificially sweetened) as a first step toward stabilizing glucose, and they also switched from refined-grain bread to whole-grain bread. They set a goal of preparing at least three "nonpackaged" meals each week, meaning no microwave or heat-and-eat dinners. They found that their meals didn't take very much time to prepare if they planned ahead and had fresh vegetables and lean-protein choices already on hand in the refrigerator. In addition to replacing soda and refined carbs with a better balance of whole grains, vegetables, and protein, Tricia and her daughters also added a daily licorice-root supplement (containing glabridin) to help further stabilize glucose levels.

After one month, Tricia's daughters found that their acne cleared up and their ability to concentrate on homework and exams was improved. Tricia herself reported a noticeable lifting of the "brain fog" that she'd been under for many months and a significant drop in her belly fat — so much so that she had to buy a smaller size of nursing scrubs.

6

Health Pillar 4 —
Balance Stress Hormones

From the very first chapter of this book, you have been learning about the effects of chronic stress, which is the main enemy of vigor. At this point, we're ready to explore the ways in which stress leads to disruptions in biochemical balance in the other three of the Four Pillars of Health (oxidation, inflammation, and glycation). Those disruptions can result in low vigor and poor health if you aren't careful to control either your *exposure* to stress or the way in which your body *responds* to stress. Before looking at what happens on the biochemical level, let's briefly review the basics of chronic stress.

Human beings were simply not meant to "carry around" constant disturbances in their stress response to the point that this response reaches the state called "chronic stress." Humans *were* built to respond to stress quickly and then to have stress hormones dissipate immediately. That is the "acute-stress" response or, as discussed in Chapter 1, "temporary" stress. When the body is exposed to wave after wave of chronic stress from the modern lifestyle, it begins to break down. Animals don't normally harbor chronic stress the way humans do, but when they do (during stress experiments, starvation, injury, etc.), they get sick just like humans do. In study after study, it quickly becomes obvious that the stress response, although helpful in certain situations, turns negative when the body begins to perceive everyday events as "stressful" events. Over time, stress-related diseases result from either an overexaggerated stress response (too much response to what should have been a small stressor) or an underexaggerated ability to shut down the stress response (which causes levels of the stress hormone cortisol to remain elevated and biochemical balance to fall apart).

Because the modern world rarely requires the evolutionary fight-or-flight response to stress, people deny their bodies their natural physical reaction to stress. Unfortunately, the brain still registers stress in the same way as it always has. But because people no longer react to that stress with vigorous physical activity (fighting or running away), the body "stores" the stress response and continues to churn out high levels of stress hormones. Before you know it, you find yourself suffering from feeling "tired/stressed/depressed" or "burnout" and feeling as if you have no control over the many stressors in your life. In one of the more ironic twists visited upon humans as "higher" animals, the brain is so "well developed" that the body has learned to respond to psychological stress with the same hormonal cascade that occurs with exposure to a physical stressor. This means that just by thinking about a stressful event, even if that event is highly unlikely to actually occur, you cause your endocrine system to get into an uproar that interferes with your biochemical balance — leading you toward burnout.

STRESS HORMONES DEFINED

A number of different biomarkers have been used in studies of chronic stress and stress-hormone balance. To help you better understand some of the concepts and vocabulary used to explain the biochemical activities that stress sets into motion, here are brief descriptions of these biomarkers:

> ❧ *Cortisol* is a hormone produced by the adrenal glands. Its main "acute" functions are to increase blood-sugar levels (via insulin antagonism), reduce inflammation, and

stimulate immune function. Its main "chronic" effects are to increase blood-sugar levels (via appetite stimulation), increase inflammation, and suppress immune function.

- *Testosterone and DHEA (dehydroepiandrosterone)* are hormones produced by the adrenal glands. They suppress inflammatory cytokines, reduce oxidative damage, and improve insulin sensitivity — but testosterone and DHEA levels are suppressed when cortisol production is elevated, so you "lose" much of their anti-inflammatory and antioxidant benefits during periods of chronic stress.

- *Epinephrine, norepinephrine,* and *dopamine* are catecholamines produced in the brain. They increase during acute stress and are involved in brain function and vigilance, but production is suppressed during chronic stress, leading to fatigue, depression, and low vigor.

- *Interleukin-6* and *TNF-alpha* are inflammatory cytokines produced by immune system cells. They normally are produced to slow acute tissue damage, but when produced chronically, they actually lead to accelerated tissue damage.

- *C-reactive protein (CRP)* is a protein synthesized in the liver. It is elevated during chronic inflammation.

STRESS HORMONES IN ACTION

When you encounter anything that causes you to feel stress, your cortisol levels go up. If you experience stressful events on a regular basis and are unable to effectively rid yourself of the stressor, then your cortisol levels stay constantly elevated. The elevation of cortisol leads to further problems with biochemical balance, such as reduced testosterone and interference with other hormones (such as insulin and thyroid hormones).

This process can be compared to what happens with a line of dominoes, where tipping one hormone off balance (cortisol) leads to a disruption in the next (testosterone) and the next (insulin) and the next (serotonin) and the next (thyroid) and so on, until eventually the balance of your entire system is upset and you feel terrible. Also lined up like dominoes are the other Pillars of Health, where cortisol excess increases levels of inflammatory cytokines, oxidative free radicals, and glycating sugars. This increase in stress-induced oxidation/inflammation is due, in part, to the fact that excess cortisol stimulates a chronic immune response that is accompanied by a "respiratory burst" from macrophages and related cells. And this response is also partly due to the increased creation of AGEs (advanced glycation end products) that is triggered by the cortisol-induced elevations in blood sugar.

Elevated cortisol levels are also associated with reduced levels of testosterone and IGF-1 in subjects exposed to high stress. (IGF-1, or insulin-like growth factor 1, is related to growth hormone.) Because testosterone and IGF-1 are anabolic, or muscle-building, hormones, the research subjects exposed to high stress also tended to have reduced muscle mass and higher body-fat levels. And they also tended to have a higher body mass index (BMI), a higher waist-to-hip ratio (WHR), and abdominal obesity (an "apple" shape). Researchers at the Neurological Institute at the University of California at San Francisco (UCSF) have linked excessive cortisol levels to depression, anxiety, and Alzheimer's disease, as well as to direct changes in brain structure (atrophy) leading to cognitive defects — meaning that cortisol can shrink and kill brain cells. All this research points to a consistent reproducible finding — that chronic stress leads to biochemical/hormonal/metabolic disruptions that put the body in a state of accelerated "breakdown" in tissues throughout it, including the brain, heart, blood vessels, muscles, bones, immune-system cells, etc. At the same time, these disruptions also suppress the "buildup" of healthy tissues, because chronic stress retards tissue growth — except for abdominal fat!

Scientific research and medical evidence clearly show that a sustained high level of cortisol — triggered by chronic, unrelenting stress and leading to a cascade of further biochemical disruptions — has debilitating effects on long-term health. Among these many effects is an increase in appetite and cravings for certain foods, especially sweets. Because one of the primary roles of cortisol is to encourage the body to refuel itself after responding to a stressor, an elevated cortisol level keeps your appetite ramped up, so you constantly feel hungry. In addition, the type of fat that accumulates as a result of this stress-induced appetite will typically locate itself in the abdominal region of the body (probably so it is readily available for release during the next stress response). The major problem with abdominal fat, aside from the fact that nobody wants a pot belly, is that this type of fat is also highly associated with increased cellular damage from glycating sugars, oxidative free radicals, and inflammatory cytokines, all of which increase the risk of developing heart disease, diabetes, and cancer.

So now you have a bit of appreciation for the challenges to biochemical balance that chronic stress causes in the body. When cortisol goes up or its normal rhythm is disrupted, a cascade of biochemical events is set into motion that disrupts other hormones, including testosterone, insulin, thyroid, and many others. Elevated cortisol also unbalances the ratio between various neurotransmitters (dopamine, norepinephrine, serotonin, and others) and other metabolic proteins (such as cytokines, which are involved in inflammation).

STRESS AND THE WELL-TRAINED ATHLETE

Stress researchers, including myself, frequently study competitive athletes. For obvious reasons, athletes are extremely interested in balancing the "dose" of stress they deliver to their bodies with the amount of recovery necessary for optimal performance. Counteracting the muscle-wasting and fat-gaining effects of prolonged cortisol exposure becomes a large part of maximizing performance gains while minimizing the risk for illness and injury. For many athletes, the delicate balance between training "stress" and recovery poses a significant dilemma: To become faster and more competitive, they have to train hard, but training too hard without adequate recovery will just make them slow, because they'll be tired or get sick or hurt. Athletes who excel at the highest levels are those who are most adept at balancing the three primary components of their programs: training, diet, and recovery. A phenomenon known as "overtraining syndrome" has been linked to chronic cortisol exposure, exactly the same situation that the average person faces in their battle with daily stressors and the struggle to maintain biochemical balance and high vigor. Although chronic overtraining is easy to recognize by its common symptoms of constant fatigue, mood fluctuations, and reduced mental and physical performance (sounds a lot like the burnout and lack of vigor suffered by many nonathletes), it may be difficult to detect in its earlier stages, just like the early stages of stress. Therefore, competitive athletes, like everyone, need to become adept at balancing exposure to stress with recovery from stress to approach the optimal physical and mental performance they are looking for.

STRESS HORMONES, DEPRESSION, AND THE LOSS OF VIGOR

Just as overexposure to certain hormones is detrimental to health, so is underexposure. Consider the effect of the primary stress hormone, cortisol, on the brain. We've known about the links between stress and depression for decades. In the United States alone, stress-related depression accounts for more than $30 billion in annual medical expenses and lost productivity. Researchers at the Institute of Psychiatry at King's College, in London, have determined that stress-related depression actually progresses in two distinct phases. The first phase is characterized by an overexposure to cortisol, creating a "toxic" effect whereby too much cortisol actually destroys crucial brain cells responsible for good mood. The second phase is a compensatory mechanism where the brain becomes resistant to the effects of cortisol as a way to "protect" itself from cortisol's damaging effects. So the brain cells (neurons) are now deprived of cortisol, creating a dramatic under-exposure that leads to a host of memory and psychological problems. Unfortunately, this syndrome of cortisol resistance leads to a deepening of depression and symptoms of fatigue and confusion, a combination that is very much like the symptoms seen in people with PTSD (post-traumatic stress disorder). A similar scenario occurs for other hormones, whereby over- or underexposure leads to a host of physical and psychological dysfunctions, which are alleviated upon restoring metabolic balance.

Remember, vigor is a measure not only of your physical health but also of your mental state and functioning. Because the over-exposure or underexposure to cortisol in the brain can destroy a good mood and lead to depression, fatigue, and confusion, you can begin to see how an imbalance in stress hormones can negatively impact your vigor.

In some respects, you can think of certain aspects of stress-hormone balance in the same way that you might think about getting too little, enough, or too much exercise. Some is good, too little is bad, and too much is bad. Overtrained athletes (who are over-stressed physically and mentally) often have low levels of cortisol during exercise (when they should be high), but high levels during rest (when they should be low). These out-of-sync cortisol levels indicate that the bodies of these athletes are still under stress and out of biochemical balance, perhaps from injury, infection, or inadequate recovery. These athletes also experience fatigue, weight gain, depressed mood, and poor performance.

Because of the close link between stress and depression, every major pharmaceutical company in the world is rushing to develop new drugs to modulate or restore biochemical balance. The current antidepressant drugs work primarily on serotonin in the brain, and some newer ones also increase norepinephrine levels, but none of them truly addresses biochemical balance in a holistic manner. This means that only about half the people who try antidepressant drugs should expect to see any relief in their depression, yet these drugs still account for approximately $20 billion in sales every year. Think back to the discussion in Chapter 4 about the folly and danger associated with trying to address the multifaceted nature of inflammation with dangerous COX-2 inhibitor drugs, and you'll have an appreciation for why antidepressant drugs are often the wrong "solution" for a multifaceted "problem," such as stress-induced burnout and depression.

Among the drug companies that are furiously trying to come up with an answer to stressed-out people with disrupted biochemical balances are Bristol-Myers Squibb, GlaxoSmithKline, Pfizer, Sanofi-Aventis, Johnson & Johnson, Merck, and Novartis. Several of these companies already make antidepressant drugs that increase serotonin levels, including Pfizer (Zoloft), Eli Lilly (Prozac and Cymbalta), Glaxo (Paxil), and Wyeth (Effexor). But because these drugs are only effective about half the time, and because they now have to carry an FDA-mandated "black box" safety warning due to their extreme side effects, including an increased risk of suicide, there are many reasons to look for a better solution to the problem of stress-related depression. A "black box" warning is a special warning that appears on the package insert for prescription drugs that may cause serious adverse effects, including severe risk of death. It gets its name from the bold black border that surrounds the text of the warning. A black box warning is the strongest warning that the FDA has and is only required for the most dangerous drugs.

BALANCE STRESS HORMONES— AND VIGOR WILL FOLLOW

Numerous studies convincingly show that reducing "biochemical stress"—including restoring balance between various measures, such as cortisol, testosterone, glucose, cytokines, CRP, and others — also reduces the risk of dying and increases lifespan. Positive changes in psychological measures of stress, such as a greater sense of "meaningfulness in life," have also been associated with improvements in biochemical balance markers. But this "psychobiochemical" effect appears to cut both ways, because individuals with "downward" financial mobility (such as job loss) tend to have higher indices of cortisol/cytokines, and those individuals with the highest financial stress (poverty) have been shown to have a striking six-year-shorter life expectancy, attributable to increased disease risk from excessive metabolic stress. In similar fashion, the risk of developing burnout, chronic fatigue syndrome (CFS), or post-traumatic stress disorder (PTSD) has recently been shown to be approximately three times higher in subjects with elevated psychological stress and dysregulations across the Four Pillars.

Numerous forms of "stress management" exist, and many fine references are available on that topic. However, this book takes the view that although stress-management techniques have been around for decades, very few of those regimens have made a large impact on the health or well-being of the average person. This fact has nothing to do with the techniques' being ineffective — they work if you can actually put them into practice. For many people, however, wedging another stress-management tool into their already busy lives does little more than just add further stress. I know that some stress-management gurus will disagree with me, but from a purely practical point of view (from my position as a nutritional biochemist and an exercise physiologist), most people can't be bothered with traditional approaches to stress management. And many rarely take the time to exercise or eat the way they know they should — both of which could go a long way toward reducing the detrimental effects of stress on the body.

Giving up old unhealthy habits — such as grabbing a fast-food meal when you're feeling stressed instead of sitting down to a nutritious dinner — is always a challenge. But besides the difficulties of changing behavior, I believe most people do not take advantage of stress busters, such as exercise or dietary supplements, simply because the idea that stress can seriously damage health has not really sunk in — including for many in the medical profession. Almost everyone is now aware that smoking is bad for you, and laws have systematically reduced the number of places where cigarette smoking is allowed. I don't think society has reached that critical mass of opinion about the impact of stress, though. In Chapter 1, I stated that I believe it is just as important to get your stress levels under control as it is to eat a healthy diet and get physical activity. Once you let that idea sink in — and once you've absorbed the information about how much damage stress can do to your heart, your brain, and your overall health — I believe you will naturally begin to adopt the behaviors that will help you balance your stress hormones.

To make it easier for you, I've outlined the best strategies for restoring balance across your personal Four Pillars of Health, and I've grouped them into several categories that I define as "Vigor Improvement Practices" (VIPs). You'll find details on these practices in the last part of this book — Part III — which I designed for people asking "what to do" to build vigor. The best thing "to do" is to take small steps, and I've intentionally kept my recommendations simple so you can easily incorporate them into your lifestyle. You should also be encouraged by the fact that thousands of clients and participants in my programs have successfully used these practices and enjoyed noticeable benefits in relatively short periods of time — without undue hardship or inconvenience in their already busy and stressful lives. I'm confident the same results are available to you.

PILLAR POINTS TO REMEMBER...

I hope that these four chapters in Part II have given you an appreciation of the importance of restoring biochemical balance within each — and between each — of the Four Pillars of Health. In some ways, it may seem that balancing stress hormones is the most important task in restoring vigor, because these hormones are the "master controllers" of your biochemistry. But, as stated throughout this book, the pillars are interdependent and intertwined with each other, so it makes sense to strengthen all of them *simultaneously* to create a truly comprehensive approach to optimal health. As with the example of the dominoes, if you make a positive change regarding one of the pillars, you will set off positive reactions in all the rest.

THE PILLARS IN ACTION (BURNOUT AND OVERTRAINING)

Michael was a lawyer and runner who Balanced Stress Hormones to beat burnout and overtraining. As an attorney specializing in intellectual-property issues (patents, trademarks, etc.), Michael worked extremely long hours at his desk, reading papers and working on his computer. He used running as his mental and physical "release" from the stresses of the day — it gave him some time to think about creative solutions to his clients' issues. As a former All-American cross-country runner in college, Michael remained highly competitive in his postcollege years and was training for an attempt at the Olympic Trials for the marathon. Unfortunately, due to the combination of the psychological stress from Michael's highly stressful career (which had become even more so due to layoffs at his law firm) and a significant increase in physical stress from his increased training load for the Olympic Trials, Michael quickly found himself having trouble concentrating at work and unmotivated to lace up his running shoes to train.

After visiting his chiropractor for some help with a slow-healing hip injury, Michael was told that his cortisol was high and his testosterone was low — and that this biochemical imbalance was likely at the root of his lack of motivation for work or running.

On his chiropractor's advice, Michael incorporated a few simple Vigor Improvement Practices to help balance his stress hormones and lead him away from burnout and back to vigor. In addition to striving for eight hours of sleep each night, especially on his hardest running days, Michael became more attuned to balancing high-stress workdays with moderate-stress training days and moderate-stress workdays with high-stress training days. As a lawyer working toward a partnership and as an Olympic hopeful, Michael typically had no "low-stress" days, but to help beat his burnout, he also agreed to have one "no-stress" day per week where he was completely "off" from work and training. In addition to these steps, Michael also added a daily eurycoma root supplement to directly restore balance between cortisol/testosterone.

Within a period of about six months, Michael improved his cortisol/testosterone balance by 30 percent and improved his Vigor Index from an extremely low level (27, associated with extreme burnout) to a very high level (4, associated with optimal physical and mental performance). His life improved — with Michael benefitting from improved mental clarity to get more work done with less stress (he made partner) and also from improved physical/mental energy, which allowed him to train and compete at a higher level (he did not qualify for the Olympic Games, but he ran a personal-best marathon time).

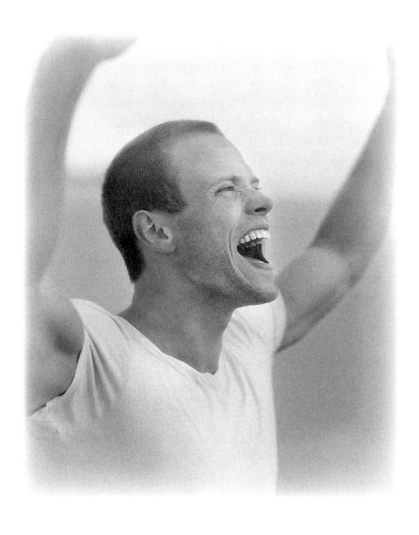

PART III [vigor improvement practices]

Whether your goal is to win the Super Bowl or just clean the toilet bowl, you need to have high vigor, and you no doubt want to feel good on a daily basis. This final section of the book focuses on the "what-to-do" aspects of restoring biochemical balance to beat burnout and bring back your vigor. The next few chapters present a range of recommendations involving sleep/stress, nutrition, exercise, and dietary supplements that have been shown to work to restore biochemical balance and help people recover their desired states of high vigor. Best of all, these recommendations—which I call the "Vigor Improvement Practices" (VIPs)—not only are effective but can also be *realistically* implemented by virtually anyone.

My recommendation: Do as many of these VIPs as you can for one week and see how much your vigor improves. I have witnessed hundreds of clients enjoy phenomenal results after only seven days of incorporating these health-promoting activities into their lives. Some people will begin by focusing on exercising and getting more sleep, while others may start by taking dietary supplements and using stress-management techniques, such as meditation. After the first week, of course, you can continue the practices that work best for you and watch your vigor improve even more. Once you have read through the information on each individual VIP, Chapter 11 helps you put it all together in a chart that you can update and adapt to your own needs.

To put it very simply, the VIPs help you achieve biochemical equilibrium in your body by restoring balance in each of the Four Pillars of Health. By establishing this biochemical balance, your body is once again able to resume its natural process of tissue repair and rejuvenation. The diet, exercise, and flexibility portions of the VIPs form the foundation that promotes healthy tissue turnover throughout the entire body. Dietary supplements provide the most concentrated source of biochemical regulators and tissue building blocks that the body needs to support optimal turnover, synthesis, and repair. The combined effect of exercise, stretching, proper nutrition, and supplements results in an ideal environment to restore biochemical balance, promote tissue health, and improve vigor.

The VIPs are not only a simple and effective approach to regaining and maintaining your vigor but a new way to think about the health of your tissues and keeping the "state of repair" in your body in optimal condition. By maintaining proper balance and function and supporting the body's vital renewal processes, the VIPs can help delay or prevent many of the degenerative conditions commonly associated with aging — including burnout, depression, arthritis, and fibromyalgia — plus many of the aches and pains that nearly everyone confronts with advancing years. The VIPs can help virtually everybody, from professional athletes to weekend warriors to never-exercisers. The main goal is for you to learn how to imbed these practices into your life *each and every day* to achieve and maintain a healthy active lifestyle — and enjoy a greater level of vigor!

7

[vigor improvement practices]

Stress Management
and Sleep

R esearch studies are quite clear on the fact that reducing
stress also reduces overall cortisol exposure and that reducing cortisol exposure is a "good thing" for your long-
term health and vigor. That's all well and good — but I also understand that *telling* you to manage stress is a lot easier than actually
controlling it in your frantic life. It might help to understand that
you're not alone in this regard (as discussed in Chapter 6). Do you
think it is a coincidence that so many Americans rate "stress" as the
number-one reason for a trip to the doctor, while medical surveys
clearly indicate that men show up most often at the doc with lower
back pain or fatigue, while women tend to report fibromyalgia or
depression? That's not a coincidence — that's direct evidence that
stressed-out lives are causing people to hurt and feel terrible! The
stress exposure that you're awash in each and every day eventually shows itself as problems with biochemical balance, possibly
manifesting as burnout and ultimately as outright tissue damage.
You need to *do* something about it. This chapter focuses on two
critical Vigor Improvement Practices (VIPs): stress management
and sleep.

Whenever I give a public seminar on stress and biochemical balance, I like to start off by holding up a glass of water and asking the audience to guess how much it weighs. People will generally call out guesses that range from six to twenty ounces. But the point I like to make is that the actual *weight* of the water glass doesn't matter. As a "stress" to my arm, the weight of the water glass is less important than the *duration* of time that I need to hold it up. If I hold the glass for a minute or two, then it is not much of a stress at all, but if you were to ask me to hold it for an hour or a day or a week, then I'd be in trouble. It works the same way with your exposure to other stressors — such as traffic, bills, family commitments, and the millions of other little stresses that you encounter day in and day out. Eventually, you will reach a breaking point unless you actively manage those stresses. *Everybody* — no matter how "tough" you think you are, no matter how "resistant" to stress you think you are, no matter how much you think that you "thrive" on stress — has a personal "breaking point" when it comes to stress exposure. By managing stress and getting adequate sleep — as well as incorporating the other VIPs, including nutrition, exercise, and dietary supplementation to restore balance in each of the Four Pillars of Health — you can continually modulate your own individual stress load and hopefully keep that "breaking point" at bay.

Okay, back to my glass of water. Let's say that I'm asked to hold the water glass for a week. Impossible, you might say. Not so — because if I'm smart about managing this stress, I might be able to handle it. Maybe I can take short breaks, where I put the glass down for a few minutes each hour. Perhaps I can lessen my personal burden by asking a colleague or a friend or family member to hold the glass for a little while. Maybe I can leave the glass at work and not worry about dragging this "burden" home with me. Any and all of these (and dozens of other) strategies are ways in which I can "manage" my stress response — even if just for a few minutes. Think about some of your own sources of stress as well as some ways that you can remove yourself from exposure to those stressors.

Consider a study by the Families and Work Institute showing that one in three American workers felt chronically overworked because of "technology" (mostly cell phones and e-mail that enable people to be working anywhere and everywhere, all the time). It is really too bad that "being busy" has become such a status symbol, because it is clear from the scientific research that being too busy and always being "on" is detrimental to long-term physical and mental health. Don't get me wrong — hard work is important and valuable, but working too hard for too long leads to burnout, reduced creativity, and inefficiency. It is not much of an overstatement to say that you can literally work yourself to death.

We know from studies of animals and humans that at least three factors can make a huge difference in how the body responds to a given stressor:

1. whether the stress has any *outlet*

2. whether the stressor is *predictable*

3. whether the human or animal thinks it has any *control* over the stressor

These three factors — outlet, predictability, and control — emerge as modulating factors again and again in research studies of stress. For example, if you put a rat in a cage and subject it to a series of low-voltage electric shocks, the rat develops metabolic imbalance and stomach ulcers (wouldn't you?). If you take another rat, give it the same series of shocks, but also give it an *outlet* for its stress — such as something to chew on, something to eat, or a wheel to run on — it is able to maintain biochemical balance and does *not* get ulcers. The same is true for humans under stress: Go for a run, scream at the wall, or do something else that serves as an outlet for maintaining metabolic balance, and you can counteract or at least modulate many of the detrimental effects of stress.

Let's turn now to the second of the three stress modulators: *predictability*. Suppose someone woke you up in the middle of the night, put you on a plane, and then made you jump out of it at ten thousand feet. Pretty stressful, huh? This experience would certainly be accompanied by elevated heart rate and blood pressure, changes in blood levels of glucose and fatty acids, and, of course, a huge disruption in biochemical balance. What do you think would happen if you were forced to do this every other night for the next few months? Far from being a stressed-out bundle of nerves, you would actually get accustomed to it—and your stress response would become less pronounced. This scenario has actually been studied in U.S. Army Rangers who were training at "jump school" to become paratroopers. At the start of training, the soldiers endured enormous increases in stress-hormone levels during each jump (indicating they were out of biochemical balance). But by the end of the course, their stress responses were virtually nonexistent. By making the stressor more *predictable* (you know it is coming, and you are prepared for it), the stress response of each soldier was controlled to a much greater degree.

Finally, the concept of *control* is central to understanding why some people respond to a stressor with gigantic disruptions in biochemical balance, while others respond to the same stressor with little more than a yawn. This idea has been demonstrated in rats that have been trained to press a lever to avoid getting shocked. Every time the rat gets shocked, it presses the lever, and the next shock is delayed for several minutes. Because the rat has some degree of control over his situation, it also has a lower occurrence of stress-related diseases (such as ulcers and infections). An interesting comparison can be made to people working under high-stress conditions, such as during a period of corporate layoffs. For many workers, this situation is one of high instability and low control (thus high stress), while others, perhaps those in a department that will be unaffected by job cuts or among people who have a "fallback" plan (such as a part-time job on the side), experience much less stress and fewer health problems.

Keep in mind that the concept of *control* does not mean that you need to try to gain a high degree of control over every aspect of your life, because trying to do so can actually increase your stress and lead to a high degree of metabolic imbalance. Instead, managing stress usually means doing your best to control those things you have the power to control and accepting those things that you have little (or no) control over.

The strategies outlined in the next section may also be useful to you in grappling with the all-important issue of stress as part of your comprehensive approach to raising your level of vigor.

[vip] STRESS-MANAGEMENT STRATEGIES

Whether you on the verge of burnout or just a little tired from a typical twenty-first-century day, the last thing you may want to hear is someone telling you to "reduce stress." I'm right there with you. Fortunately, a multitude of effective strategies for managing stress are available to you; best of all, you do not have to drastically alter your lifestyle to implement most of them. These ideas for managing stress are backed up by research that shows they can be extremely effective. Here are a few of my favorites that I have shared with clients and readers over the years, and I invite you to consider incorporating them into your daily routine to build vigor.

Manage your electronic interruptions. The beeps, buzzes, or other sounds from your computer (not to mention those from an iPhone, Blackberry, or whatever new devices come on the market by the time you read this) can add an annoying level of stress to your day. Instead of just responding every time you get an electronic interruption, take charge of those devices and set them to only alert you at specific times. For instance, most e-mail programs are automatically set to check for new messages every five minutes (which means you're interrupted by the "new-message beep" ninety-six times in an eight-hour day!). How do you expect to get any "real" work done? Also, consider (as I do) shutting off your e-mail program until the second half of your day, enabling you to get your "important" work accomplished in the morning when you're mentally fresh.

Whenever possible, leave the cell phone behind. It may be hard to imagine today, but it wasn't too many years ago that people got along perfectly fine without cell phones. Try taking a break from your phone when possible by leaving it behind. I make that recommendation, because if you carry your phone with you — even if you tell yourself that you won't answer it — a part of your mind still waits for it to ring (or buzz, or play your favorite ring-tone). Let that part of your brain relax and forget about the phone every now and then.

Read trash. Get a book or magazine that has no redeeming social value — and enjoy it. If this is too decadent for your tastes, then alternate a "good" book that might teach you something with a "junk" book that you can simply lose yourself in. Why? Because it allows your mind to "escape" and recharge so it comes back even stronger, more creative, and more resilient to stress. Once, on a cross-country flight, I sat next to a woman who was reading a ge-netic research journal. (I was reading a bicycling magazine.) As a fellow scientist, I commented on her reading material, and she laughed, because underneath her research journal she had one of those celebrity-gossip tabloids that you see at the grocery check-out stand. She explained that she couldn't wait to "get through" her genetics journal so she could "catch up" on the latest "dirt" — it was hilarious. It turns out that we were both headed to the same obesity-research conference in Boston, and we both appreciated the importance of "getting away" for a few minutes in our "junky" books and magazines.

Take a mini-vacation every day. One of the best ways to de-stress during your workday is to revive the lost art of lunch. Take it! Too may people skip lunch (bad metabolically and mentally) or gobble it down at their desks (which is even worse). Instead, take the hour to enjoy a healthy meal and relax your mind. Even bet-ter, use that hour to visit with friends or coworkers — you'll have a more productive second half of the day and likely accomplish even more high-quality work with improved creativity and efficiency than if you had worked through lunch. And be sure to get up from your desk every hour or two for a quick stretch or walk around the office. You'll be amazed at how a quick flex of your muscles and a surge in your circulation can help clear the cobwebs from your mind.

Take a full day off each week. No work. No thoughts about work or worries about work. Take this day to relax, reflect, and recharge (regardless of whether or not a "Sabbath" day of rest has any religious connotations for you). Read a book. Take a walk. Luxuriate in the act of doing nothing. I guarantee that if you give yourself over to a solid month of "do-nothing Sundays" (or Satur-days, or whichever day of the week works for your schedule), you will feel more physically and mentally refreshed than you could possibly imagine. Doing nothing will give you back a lot.

Recreate to re-create. Giving yourself permission to relax does not mean that you're a slacker; it means that you're a step ahead of the nose-to-the-grindstone automatons who are on a fast road to burnout. As a long-time nutrition consultant to some very elite-level athletes, I can tell you without question that knowing when to "go hard" and when to "ease off" is what separates Olympic champions from also-rans. Although your own life might be "too busy" most of the time, it is those moments of relaxation and de-compression that allow you to keep jumping back in with renewed energy and creativity.

Get a massage or take a bath. Australian researchers have shown that something as simple as a fifteen-minute weekly back massage reduced cortisol levels (restoring metabolic balance), blood pressure, and overall measures of anxiety in a group of high-stress nurses. Another study of massage conducted at the University of Miami School of Medicine showed a remarkable 31 percent reduction in cortisol levels following massage therapy, as well as a 28 percent increase in the feel-good neurotransmitter serotonin. In similar studies, Japanese scientists in Osaka have shown a significant reduction in cortisol levels in high-stress men following relaxing hot baths. The men with the highest stress levels had the most dramatic reductions in cortisol levels. These studies prove that the relaxing nature of massage and hot baths is an effective approach to maintaining biochemical balance.

Imagine creative solutions. Japanese researchers in Kyoto have shown that guided-imagery exercises (relaxing by imagining solutions to stress) can help people maintain biochemical balance after the very first session. In a series of studies, subjects practiced replacing unpleasant mental images of stressful events with comfortable thoughts, resulting in a displacement of stress, a shift toward a balanced emotional state, and a significant restoration of biochemical balance. Psychology researchers at UCLA have also shown that stressed patients who performed a "value-affirmation task" (mentally reciting their personal values and itemizing the things that were most important to them) in reaction to stressful events were able to maintain biochemical balance even under these circumstances.

Believe in yourself. Remember the story of *The Little Engine Who Could*? Well, young children show marked resilience to stress when they apply the same "I think I can" approach to school stressors as the little train did in its attempt to climb the hill in the classic tale. In a study by Swedish researchers, school kids had reduced stress responses and were better able to maintain biochemical balance when they approached stressful situations with mental imagery that affirmed, "I can solve this task."

Get away for a long weekend. Even short periods of "getting away" can result in a significant drop in cortisol levels. In one study, a three-day, two-night weekend resulted in a decrease in cortisol levels and overall stress markers (indicating a restoration of biochemical balance) as well as a boost in immune-system function.

Take a yoga class. Swedish psychologists have recently shown that ten sessions of yoga over four weeks resulted in significant psychological and physiological benefits in men and women. Participants in the yoga sessions showed improvements in their levels of cortisol, stress, anger, exhaustion, and blood pressure.

Pray. Regardless of how you feel about religion or spirituality, research shows that prayer can have an impact on health. One study on religion by researchers at Arizona State University has shown that people who are more spiritual and pray more often have lower cortisol levels and lower blood pressure.

Get a pet. For some people, stress management may come on four legs. Scientists at Virginia Commonwealth University found that high-stress health-care professionals were able to significantly lower their cortisol levels after as little as five minutes of "dog therapy." (Although no one measured the biochemical balance in the pooches, it is quite possible that they also benefited from playing with the health-care workers.)

Tune in to tunes. Listening to relaxing music (as compared to sitting in silence) can significantly reduce cortisol levels following a stressful event, according to studies by French scientists.

Get some sleep. Easily the *most* effective stress-management technique you can practice is really very simple: Get enough sleep. Even one or two nights of good, sound, restful sleep can do more for maintaining your biochemical balance and reducing your long-term risk for many chronic diseases than a whole lifetime of stress-management classes. It is almost impossible to overstate the crucial role adequate sleep plays in controlling your stress response, helping you to lose weight, boosting your energy levels, improving your mood, and, of course, raising your level of vigor.

Because sleep is such an important component for building vigor, I'm devoting the rest of the chapter to it.

THE IMPORTANCE OF GETTING ENOUGH SLEEP

Just as you pay little attention to the fact that your heart beats in a regular pattern, so too are you normally unaware of your body's natural rhythm during restful sleep. But night after night, your body follows a well-worn path into dreamland: Breathing slows, muscles relax, heart rate and blood pressure drop, and body temperature falls. The brain releases the "sleep hormone," melatonin, and begins a slow descent into sleep. The rapid beta waves of your restless wakeful state in the daytime gradually change into the slower alpha waves that are characteristic of calm wakefulness, or "relaxed alertness," where you generally want to spend most of your time. Eventually, your brain drops into the still-slower theta waves that predominate during the various stages of sleep. During a full night of sleep, you normally pass through several stages: Stage 2 (lasting ten to fifteen minutes), then Stage 3 (lasting five to fifteen minutes), and finally to the deepest portion of sleep in Stage 4 (lasting about thirty minutes). Even though Stage 4 lasts only about a half hour, it is the most "famous" portion of the sleep cycle, because it is when you dream and exhibit rapid eye movement, popularly referred to as REM. Your total sleep cycle, from early Stage 2 to final REM sleep, takes an average of ninety minutes to complete. And, most importantly for people who have trouble sleeping, this cycle repeats itself over and over throughout the night — which means that interruptions can make it harder to get back to sleep, depending on which part of the cycle the sleeper is experiencing when awakened. In sleep-research labs, where alarm clocks, lights, and other interruptions can be banished, scientists have found that the natural duration of these repeating sleep cycles (the "physiological ideal") is eight hours and fifteen minutes.

The idea of getting more than eight hours of sleep per night may sound great — but what if you simply can't (or won't) get that much shut-eye? You could be setting yourself up for numerous health problems, beginning with the fact that your blood-sugar levels will rise. Sleep researchers have shown that getting only four to six hours of sleep per night results in signs of impaired glucose tolerance and insulin resistance. This means that cheating on sleep — even for only a few nights — can put a person in a prediabetic state. These changes in insulin action and blood-sugar control are also linked to the development of obesity and an increase in risk for inflammation-related conditions, such as heart disease. Poor sleep also contributes to obesity, because it precipitates changes on the hormonal level. Growth hormone and leptin are reduced in people who spend less time in deep sleep. (Leptin is a hormone that plays important roles in regulating appetite, body weight, metabolism, and reproductive function.) When you have less growth hormone in your system, it typically results in a loss of muscle and a gain of fat over time. Reduced levels of leptin will lead to hunger and carbohydrate cravings.

Given all these health impacts, I am continually astonished by how many people think they can just "get by" with inadequate sleep and are then surprised when they struggle with low energy, weight gain, constant hunger, depression, or any of the other problems associated with being "out" of biochemical balance. Thinking that you can "get by" with inadequate sleep is exactly like thinking you can "get by" with a steady diet of Twinkies. If you're "shorting" yourself on sleep, you are virtually guaranteeing that your biochemical balance will be chronically disrupted, and you are putting yourself in a position of weakness in each of the Four Pillars of Health.

To give you some idea of just how detrimental a lack of sleep can be to your biochemical balance, look at what happens to an average fifty-year-old who sleeps just six hours per night. That middle-aged person has nighttime cortisol levels more than *twelve* times higher than the average thirty-year-old who sleeps eight hours per night! Not only will an inadequate quality or quantity of sleep upset biochemical balance, but it will also limit your ability to fall asleep the next night (because your cortisol is still too high) and the amount of time that your mind spends in the most restful stages of deep sleep. A vicious cycle gets set into motion when you experience poor sleep, an overactive stress response, and subtle changes in biochemical balance that lead you down the path toward burnout and chronic diseases.

Numerous research studies verify the damage caused by sleep deprivation, including the following:

* A Yale University study of 1,709 men found that those who regularly got less than six hours of shut-eye *doubled* their risk of weight gain and diabetes because of elevated cortisol and its interference with insulin metabolism and blood-sugar control (leading to glycation).

* University of Virginia researchers have reported that jet lag — and the elevated cortisol that comes from sleep deprivation and altered body-clock cycles — is not just bad for health but can lead to higher death rates as well (at least in older mice). The increased death rates are thought to be due to a suppression of immune-system function by disrupted biochemical balance. The fact that these sleep-deprived mice die sooner probably comes as no surprise to exhausted, globe-trotting business executives or stretched-to-the-limit soccer moms.

* Researchers at Brown University Medical School have also shown that sleep *quality* (how restful your sleep is), but not necessarily sleep *quantity* (how many hours of sleep

you get), is closely related to biochemical balance and your state of vigor. As you might imagine, subjects with lower levels of sleep quality (including children and teenagers) also had the most disrupted biochemical balance and overall stress, as well as the lowest vigor scores.

❦ In Stockholm, Sweden, researchers at the National Institute for Psychosocial Medicine conducted a series of experiments related to those at Brown and showed that total sleep time was significantly decreased (leading to problems with biochemical balance) in workers during their most stressful workweeks. The stress at work also led to daytime sleepiness and nighttime restlessness — so even though the workers were tired, they were still too stressed and metabolically imbalanced to sleep.

Even if you understand the importance of sleep as proven in these studies, you may feel lucky to get just six or seven hours of shut-eye. I know I do — and yet I also realize this is still not enough sleep to maintain my own biochemical balance within healthy parameters. On top of that, I also know that some of the best ways to ensure a restful night of sleep are to avoid caffeine after noon (yet I sit here writing this with an afternoon cup of java next to the laptop), leave work at the office (yet I'm writing this from my home office), and skip the late-night TV (yet my DVR lets me watch primetime shows after my wife and I put the kids to bed) — so that's three strikes for me. I tell you all this "personal information" in the hope that you will see that maintaining your biochemical balance — or improving your vigor — is not an "all-or-nothing" proposition. No one does this perfectly, myself included. Sometimes you have lots of stress, and sometimes you have less. Sometimes you get adequate sleep, but for many of you, that doesn't happen often enough. On certain days you'll be able to exercise and eat right — and on other days you'll hit the drive-through and feel like you're working nonstop. The point here is not to strive to be "perfect" in your efforts to maintain biochemical balance. Rather, the best approach is to apply the principles outlined in this book as consistently as possible to ensure that you can do as much as possible to keep your vigor high as often as possible.

So I offer you the several ideas in the following section on developing better sleep habits not to give you more things to add to your "to-do" list but to present some ideas and techniques that have proven helpful to many people, including me. (Additional tips can be found at http://www.nhlbi.nih.gov/health/public /sleep/healthysleepfs.pdf). Don't feel like you need to incorporate all these ideas perfectly. Rather, these are some suggestions for you to consider and adapt to your individual needs so you can tap into one of the most powerful VIPs — getting good sleep!

[vip] BUILDING BETTER SLEEP HABITS

❋ *Exercise on a regular basis.* As indicated in earlier sections, exercise can help you reduce inflammation, stress hormones, blood sugar, and oxidation, and the pleasant postexercise fatigue may be just what you need to help you sink into your bed in the evening.

❋ *Don't exercise too close to bedtime.* Exercising too close to bedtime can increase alertness enough in some people to interfere with their ability to fall asleep.

❋ *Relax before bed.* Take time to unwind by enjoying a non-electronic relaxing activity, such as reading. Electronics, including computers, video games, and televisions, can increase alertness and stimulate the brain into a wakeful state that can make it hard to fall asleep.

❋ *Make your bedroom dark and cool.* The slow drop in body temperature that you experience in a cool room can help you feel sleepy, and a darkened room with as little light distraction as possible can help you stay asleep.

❧ *If you can't fall asleep after twenty minutes, get up.* If you try to fall asleep and can't, get up and do something relaxing, such as reading, until you feel tired enough to fall asleep. The stress that comes from trying to "force" yourself to fall asleep will almost certainly keep you awake longer and may interfere with restful sleep when you finally do drift off.

Smiling on Stress

Over the years, I have picked up a few witty sayings and anecdotes about coping with stress from friends and colleagues. I hope a few of them give you a chuckle, because laughter is a great way to ease stress:

1. Accept that some days you're the pigeon, and some days you're the statue.
2. Always keep your words soft and sweet, just in case you have to eat them.
3. If you can't be kind, at least have the decency to be vague.
4. Never put both feet in your mouth at the same time, because then you won't have a leg to stand on.
5. Nobody cares if you can't dance well. Just get up and dance.
6. Because it is the early worm that gets eaten by the bird, sleep late.
7. The second mouse gets the cheese.
8. You may be only one person in the world, but you may also be the world to one person.
9. A truly happy person is one who can enjoy the scenery on a detour.
10. We could learn a lot from crayons. Some are sharp, some are pretty, and some are dull. Some have weird names, and all are different colors, but they all have to live in the same box.

8

[vigor improvement practices]

Nutrition

When it comes to restoring biochemical balance and improving vigor, nutrition plays a key role. A proper diet offers numerous benefits, such as modulating inflammation and promoting tissue repair. It only takes a few minutes of watching television, reading magazines, or surfing the Internet, however, to see that in the United States, people have a very wide range of opinions, programs, and "experts" telling them what a "proper" diet is. Unfortunately, this barrage of information (and misinformation) causes many people to become stressed out about their diets — and when they do, it causes problems. For example, Canadian nutrition researchers have shown that "dieting" itself is a potent trigger for increasing cortisol and reducing bone mass. (In their studies, of course, "dieting" is labeled "cognitive dietary restraint" [CDR] and defined as "a perceived ongoing effort to limit dietary intake to manage body weight.") Further, researchers at Texas Tech University have reported that disrupted biochemical balance has a direct and rapid detrimental effect on health, increasing rates of breakdown in virtually every tissue in the body.

Rather than becoming stressed out about your diet, it may be more helpful to realize that making wise nutritional choices can significantly improve the way you feel, function, and perform on many levels. Those benefits can be enjoyed when you simply select a blend of nutrients from among a few certain foods, including brightly colored fruits and vegetables, teamed with whole grains and lean cuts of meat, poultry, and fish. Or instead of thinking about "dieting," look at it this way: Your diet truly "fuels" your vigor by maintaining your biochemical balance. For example, a balanced breakfast of a scrambled egg, a piece of whole-grain toast, and a glass of orange juice provides a powerful dose of antistress and biochemistry-balancing nutrients. It contains protein (in the egg), carbohydrates (in the toast and juice), B-complex vitamins (in the toast), antioxidants (in the juice), and phytonutrients (carotenoids in the egg, flavonoids in the juice, and lignans in the toast).

In reality, many people are not practicing what has been preached about good health. No matter how many times you've heard commercials reminding you to eat several servings of fruits and vegetables each day, it turns out that about 90 percent of North Americans do not eat enough fruits and veggies. As a result, more than ninety million people suffer chronic diseases. According to the Centers for Disease Control and Prevention, the most popular "vegetable" in the United States is the french fry, and of the limited produce that people do eat, nearly 80 percent comes in the form of lettuce, potatoes, corn, and peas. The Institute of Medicine (IOM), Department of Agriculture (USDA), and Department of Health and Human Services (HHS) all want Americans to eat more fruits and veggies, because scientific research shows that "more is better" in terms of overall biochemical balance and the risk for obesity, diabetes, osteoporosis, stroke, heart disease, and many cancers. To give you an example of how much "more" produce you should eat than the typical American gets, a forty-year-old man or woman should eat two and a half cups of vegetables and one and a half cups of fruit daily.

If you'd like to get more of those fruits and vegetables into your diet, you may be wondering where to start. Actually, "any" of these foods are better than "none," but those that are darker colored (dark green, dark blue/purple, bright orange, bright red, bright yellow, etc.) tend to be better sources of vitamins, minerals, and phytonutrients. Phytonutrients are specialized vitamin-like compounds found in plants ("phyto" means "plant") that provide numerous health benefits. In general, the brighter in color the fruit or vegetable, the higher the content of particular phytonutrients. For example, lycopene, a red carotenoid, is found at high levels in tomatoes, while another carotenoid, beta-carotene, is responsible for the orange color of carrots and sweet potatoes. To maximize your intake of phytonutrients and other micronutrients, try this simple (and fun) approach: "Color" your diet by trying to eat as many different colored fruits and vegetables as possible. Each day, see if you can get five different colors into your diet: one serving each that is red (tomato), blue or purple (berries), yellow (melon), orange (carrot), and green (broccoli) — or whatever colors you can find. (Note: French fries do not count as a yellow vegetable.)

Beyond fruits and vegetables, you may also be confused about "macronutrients," which are carbohydrates, protein, and fat. Many dieticians and nutritionists forget the concept of "balance" and guide their clients toward diets high in complex carbohydrates. Although it is true that most people can increase the amount of *complex* carbohydrates they eat, it is important to balance those carbohydrates with proper amounts of protein, fat, and fiber. Because we're on the subject of carbohydrates, here are a few things to keep in mind: During anxious or highly stressful times, you may even *crave* carbohydrates, such as bread and sweets. Those cravings are due in part to the effect that the stress hormone cortisol has on the body in terms of suppressing insulin function, increasing blood-sugar levels, and stimulating appetite. Your brain may also urge you to eat more carbohydrates, because they can act as a "tranquilizer" of sorts by increasing brain levels of serotonin (the neurotransmitter that calms you down). Unfortunately, although caving into the craving for carbs may give you a euphoric feeling for a few minutes, you'll surely pay for it later in the form of low energy levels, mood swings, more cravings, a tendency toward weight gain — and, of course, a loss of vigor.

Besides the problem of balancing complex carbohydrates with appropriate amounts of protein, fat, and fiber, another issue causes confusion for many people. Some popular dietary experts promote the idea that proteins are "good" and carbohydrates are "bad." Those following such misguided advice may end up consuming too much protein and not enough carbohydrates. Again, this type of approach misses the point that what you want to strive for is the right *balance* of each. Achieving this balance is of key importance, because each of the macronutrients performs a different role in the body. Protein can be thought of as the primary tissue builder (and rebuilder), because it helps you maintain lean muscle mass. But if you consume more protein than you need (as might happen when drinking some of the very high protein bodybuilding drink mixes), the result can be dehydration and bloating. By the same token, it is vital to consume carbohydrates, because they serve as the primary fuel for the brain (which cannot use any other fuel source as efficiently) and also play a role as a metabolic enhancer to encourage the body to use fat as a fuel source. A popular saying among metabolic physiologists is that "fat burns in the flame of carbohydrate," which means that the breakdown products of carbohydrate metabolism are required for the optimal breakdown of stored body fat and the conversion of that fat into energy. Finally, in addition to proteins and carbohydrates, fat and fiber are also essential to good health. They are needed to round out the balanced macronutrient mix, because they work to slow digestion and absorption of carbohydrates, control blood-sugar levels, and induce satiety (feelings of fullness). Then, too, certain kinds of dietary fat provide your only sources of the essential fatty acids (EFAs), linoleic acid and linolenic acid. These EFAs have been shown to help lower cholesterol and blood pressure; reduce the risk of heart disease, stroke, and possibly some kinds of cancer; and prevent dry hair and skin. As you can see, your body needs all the macronutrients, and it is much better to take a balanced approach to nutrition than to try to eliminate certain foods or restrict your diet in unhealthy ways.

WHAT TO AVOID?

When it comes to diet, biochemical balance, and tissue health, researchers know a great deal about what *not* to do. This comes down to avoiding or limiting your intake of highly refined carbohydrates, sodas, and processed foods containing high-fructose corn syrup and trans-fat (usually listed on the label as "hydrogenated" or "partially hydrogenated" oil). Why do you need to avoid these types of highly processed foods? Because they set off a biochemical chain reaction in the body that leads to unhealthy elevations in blood sugar, insulin, cortisol, cytokines, and free radicals — yikes! All that from eating a Twinkie!

These biochemical events are not only bad for your long-term health but also bad for your long- and short-term ability to heal and rebuild tissues. For example, chugging a sugary soda leads to microscopic tissue destruction via a number of the following related events:

* Spiking blood sugar and insulin levels lead to protein glycation and destruction of collagen and elastin (key structural proteins in healthy connective tissues).

* Elevated cortisol levels lead to imbalances in the inflammatory process in favor of proinflammatory cytokines (which lead to further tissue damage).

* Inflammatory cytokine signaling elevates free-radical destruction of tissue membranes throughout the body.

And, as you now know, all these events are detrimental to your level of vigor.

WHAT TO EAT?

The proposition that poor dietary choices can lead to so much destructive metabolism in your body is scary. However, people make these choices many times a day when they eat. Very good scientific evidence helps people choose diets that provide ingredients that not only reduce these detrimental biochemical chain reactions but also prevent and reverse the effects of oxidation, glycation, inflammation, and all the rest of the negative factors on connective tissue health.

Some of the easiest routes to controlling these metabolic marauders are the following:

- Eat more healthy (omega-3) fats and fewer unhealthy omega-6 fats.
- Eat fewer refined carbohydrates and more whole-grain carbs.
- Eat more antioxidants from brightly colored fruits/veggies and supplements.
- Reduce stress or control your exposure to the stress hormone cortisol.

GOOD FAT—GOOD CARBS

Based on data collected since the mid-1970s on more than ninety thousand women and fifty thousand men, researchers at Harvard University have shown quite convincingly that the type of fat and the type of carbohydrate that you eat are vitally important in determining your overall level of systemic inflammation and heart disease. Their recommendations focus your dietary choices toward healthy fats (olive, canola, sunflower, soy, peanut, and corn oils) and healthy carbohydrates (whole-grain foods, such as whole-wheat bread, oatmeal, and brown rice) and are associated with a 30 to 40 percent reduction in risk for inflammatory heart disease. In support of the Harvard recommendations is a 2001 study from Dutch researchers published in the *American Journal of Clinical Nutrition,* which showed that eating more monounsaturated oils was associated with better hydration of tissues (which tend to have a high water content when healthy). Researchers from the University of Colorado have also noted in the *Archives of Dermatology* the astonishing differences in rates of connective tissue (skin) inflammation between populations eating a high intake of refined carbohydrates (lots of inflammation and high rates of inflammatory conditions) compared to populations eating fewer refined carbs (very low rates of both).

Modern diets supply roughly twenty to twenty-five times more "omega-6" fatty acids as "omega-3" fatty acids — a situation that predisposes you toward proinflammatory cytokines and systemic inflammation in your body. The best way to address these imbalances is to limit your intake of omega-6 fats (especially fried foods) and increase your consumption of fatty fish, such as salmon, tuna, mackerel, and bluefish (which are high in omega-3 fats). For people who can't or don't want to eat more fatty fish, a daily essential fatty acid (EFA) supplement can provide omega-3s to help quell inflammatory cytokines. A number of studies have shown that dietary omega-3 fatty acids, because of their anti-inflammatory properties, can help modulate connective-tissue inflammation.

As you can see, just as you *are* what you eat, you also tend to *feel like* what you eat. And who wants to feel like junk? The solution, as outlined above, is to face the nutritional facts and eat your way to biochemical balance and vigor by focusing on healthy carbohydrates and fats, controlling stress and cortisol, and getting enough antioxidants and omega-3 fatty acids into your daily diet.

[vip] THE HELPING-HAND APPROACH TO EATING

Over years of working with countless people, I have developed an approach to eating that is designed to be as easy and low stress as possible. I call this method the "Helping Hand" — a simplified approach to choosing foods that involves no "counting" of calories, fat grams, or carbohydrates. Instead of all those calculations, you learn to balance your intake of carbohydrates, protein, fat, and fiber in a way that considers the *quantity* of food and, even more importantly, the *quality* of those foods. Specifically, quality refers to *what* you eat, and quantity refers to *how much* you eat. With this approach, you do not have to stick to eating only certain items from a long list of "approved" foods (because all foods are fair game), and you also don't have to worry about avoiding other foods on some "banned" list (because no foods are prohibited). Below you'll see the details on this approach, which I have used with thousands of clients and shared with readers in my other books. Here's how it works.

✤ Quality: What to Eat

Step 1 — Consider Carbohydrates
General rule: Foods that are more "whole" (in their natural, unprocessed state) are preferred choices.
Carbohydrates are not "bad" in and of themselves, but the *form* of carbohydrate that you choose will determine your body's biochemical response and your likelihood of being able to effectively control inflammation and repair/rebuild damaged tissues. Here are some examples of this principle in action:

> ✤ A whole apple is less processed than applesauce, which is less processed than apple juice — so the apple is the best choice, the applesauce is moderate, and the apple juice is least preferred. In general, all whole fruits and vegetables are "good" choices.

❧ Whole-grain forms of high-carbohydrate foods are always preferred over forms that use highly refined grains. (Think "whole grain" or "whole wheat" instead of Wonder Bread.) When choosing breads, pastas, and crackers, always look at the ingredients list for "whole-grain flour" or "whole-wheat flour" instead of products that simply state "wheat flour," which indicates a more highly refined product rather than a whole-grain product.

❧ When you can't look at a label (such as when eating out), choose grain products that are thicker, chewier, and heartier — such as "peasant breads," with added seeds, nuts, and fruits — rather than "fluffier" and "softer" breads, which indicate highly refined grains.

❧ Step 2 — Provide Protein

General rule: Any form of lean protein can be used to "complete" a refined carbohydrate.

Protein and carbs are the "yin and yang" of nutrition: They have to be consumed together for proper dietary balance (which falls apart when either one is excluded or inappropriately restricted).

❧ Leaner sources of protein are always a better choice than fattier cuts (choose 96 percent lean ground beef instead of 85 percent lean).

❧ A bagel for breakfast is not necessarily a "bad" carbohydrate, but it is not the best choice, especially if it is made from refined, white flour instead of whole-wheat flour. Your bagel can be made "better" from a biochemical standpoint by adding some protein — perhaps in the form of smoked salmon or a scrambled egg. The combination of virtually any protein with a refined-carb food balances the meal into one with a better overall metabolic profile, meaning that your body will handle the calories more appropriately.

Step 3 — Finish with Fat

General rule: A small amount of added fat at each meal is a "metabolic regulator."

A bit of added fat—in the form of a pat of butter, a dash of olive oil, a square of cheese, or a small handful of nuts—helps slow the postmeal metabolic imbalance (that is, a rise in cortisol and blood sugar), which in turn helps you control appetite and enhance fat burning throughout the day.

* Your choice of pasta as a side dish (but not as a main meal—see quantity discussion in the next section) is an "okay" choice, but you can make it a better choice by selecting whole-grain pasta (instead of the typical highly refined forms) and by topping it with a delicious olive oil, garlic, and basil sauce. Even better, mix some fresh vegetables into the sauce to further boost the nutritional content of the entire meal.

* Your child's lunch of white bread with grape jelly is a biochemical disaster (you might as well inject sugar straight into her veins and fat into her adipose tissue), but you can boost the nutritional content and her body's ability to metabolize her sandwich by adding a bit of peanut butter, insisting that she wash it down with a glass of skim or 1 percent milk, and switching to whole-wheat bread (a tough switch with many kids, but well worth the try).

Step 4 — Fill Up with Fiber

General rule: Choosing "whole" forms of grains, fruits, and vegetables (as recommended in Step 1) will automatically satisfy your fiber needs.

Like fat, fiber helps slow the absorption of sugar from the digestive tract into the bloodstream. In this way, fiber can also be considered a "metabolic regulator" to help balance cortisol and blood-sugar levels at each meal or snack. The fiber content of whole foods also provides a great deal of "satiety" — that is, foods high in fiber make you feel fuller for longer, so you are less likely to feel hungry and less likely to feel stressed out as a result of your hunger. Whole-grain, fiber-rich foods also contain a wide array of antioxidant and anti-inflammatory phytonutrients, such as lignans, to further protect tissues from damage.

❧ Quantity: How Much to Eat—The "Helping-Hand" Approach to Eating

At the same time that you are evaluating the *quality* aspects of your food choices, you should also be considering the second part of the nutrition equation: *quantity* (otherwise known as "portion control"). If you look at the graphics involved with the Helping-Hand approach, you see four images:

1. a wide-open hand (representing fruits/vegetables)
2. a closed fist (concentrated carbohydrates, or starches)
3. a palm (protein)
4. an "OK" sign (added fat)

These graphics are a simple way to help you visualize controlling the "quantity" part of your diet without really "counting" calories. They also help you remember to eat an appropriate amount of food to restore biochemical balance and improve vigor. The Helping Hand works like this:

Fruits and Vegetables (except potatoes, which count as concentrated carbs, or "starches")
Choose a quantity of fruits and vegetables that roughly matches the size of your open hand. Select brightly colored fruits and vegetables for the highest levels of disease-fighting carotenoids (orange, red, yellow) and flavonoids (green, blue, purple).

Carbohydrates — Two Types

General rule: Whenever possible, select "whole" and "least processed" carbohydrate sources — but only eat a certain quantity of them (a "fist-sized" or "hand-sized" amount, as shown to the left).

Starches (such as bread, cereal, pasta, and other "concentrated" carbohydrate sources, including potatoes and potato products like french fries)

Choose a quantity that is no larger than your tightly closed fist (a small side dish of pasta, potato salad, a dinner roll, etc.).

Protein

General rule: Whenever possible, avoid consuming carbohydrates (whether whole-grain or refined) without added protein.

Lean proteins, such as eggs, low-fat yogurt, low-fat milk, lean ground beef, steak (with visible fat trimmed), fish (any), chicken, pork chops, etc. should be consumed in an amount that approximately matches the size of the palm of your hand. (Note that I said *palm* — I am not referring to your entire open hand.) Keep in mind that this portion is likely to be only about half the standard portion served in many restaurants — so be prepared to eat half and bring the other half home for leftovers.

Fat

General rule: Whenever possible, avoid consuming carbohydrates (whether whole-grain or refined) without added fat.

Any source of fat will do — butter, olive oil, flaxseed oil, canola oil, cheese, and nuts are fine. Make an "okay" sign with your thumb and index finger, and choose an amount of fat about the size of the circle formed by your index finger/thumb.

As you can see, the Helping Hand approach to eating requires zero counting of calories, fat grams, or carb grams. Why? Because the calorie control is already "built in," based on the size of your hands — think of them as Mother Nature's automatic portion control. If you have average-sized hands (and likely an average-sized body and metabolism), you will consume about five hundred calories from each meal based on this approach. Smaller individuals (with smaller hands and metabolic rates) will have smaller meals with approximately four hundred calories each; while larger people (with larger hands and metabolic rates) will have larger meals that come closer to six hundred calories each. Eat this way at breakfast, lunch, and dinner, and you'll consume about twelve hundred to eighteen hundred calories over the course of the day — or precisely the same range of calories associated with the very best programs for successfully maintaining biochemical balance, vigor, and body weight over the long term.

9

[vigor improvement practices]

Exercise

Participating in moderate exercise on a regular basis can reduce body fat, build muscle and bone, improve mental and
emotional function, stimulate the immune response, and
reduce appetite. Being physically active can also offset some of the
destructive effects of chronic stress and help restore biochemical
balance — which leads to more vigor. No drug can do all that! In
terms of improving your general sense of well-being, exercise gen-
erates the production of dopamine and serotonin, both of which
are "feel-good" anti-anxiety and antidepression chemicals that
are produced in the brain and are responsible for the well-known
"runner's high" that can help control the stress response.

Here are a few research findings that attest to the astounding
benefits of exercise:

- Duke University researchers have reported that exercise
  (thirty minutes per day, three to four days a week, for four
  months) is more effective than prescription antidepres-
  sants in relieving symptoms of anxiety and depression.

- Several studies at the University of Colorado have shown
  how exercise can reduce many of the detrimental effects of

chronic stress. The Colorado researchers also reported that *extremes* of exercise, such as regimens undertaken by over-trained endurance athletes, can *reverse* these health benefits by upsetting biochemical balance. Going to extremes with an exercise regimen caused an increase in cortisol and also suppressed testosterone in male and female athletes, biochemical effects that can quickly lead to increased body fat, interference with mental and emotional function, suppressed immune function, and a higher risk of injury.

❋ Scientists at the National Institutes of Health have noted that regular exercise can help patients with Cushing's syndrome — a condition caused by extreme disruptions in biochemical balance — to prevent much of the tissue destruction normally seen during the course of the disease.

❋ In Arizona, stress researchers reported that being more physically fit had a protective effect against feelings of stress and age-related disruptions in biochemical balance. The research findings demonstrated that less physically fit women had significantly greater problems with biochemical balance in response to stressful events compared to physically fit women.

One of the most important factors when it comes to exercise is your purpose for doing it: The "reason" you should be physically active has less to do with directly burning calories and losing weight (although those may be nice side benefits) and more to do with the fact that exercise can act as a "hedge" against the tendency for stress, sleep deprivation, aging, and poor diet to upset the body's biochemical balance. Many people tend to overestimate the rate at which exercise can burn calories. They fail to realize that you would have to run a *half mile* to burn off every Oreo you eat and almost *90 minutes* to burn off the calories in a Big Mac! So although it is true that exercise does burn calories, its primary value as part of your strategy for improving vigor lies in its profound effects on restoring biochemical balance by modulating levels of cortisol, testosterone, growth hormone, serotonin, and other biochemical compounds in the Four Pillars of Health.

You might be wondering whether a "best" type of exercise will improve biochemical balance. In reality, the best form of exercise is *anything*—as long as you do it! You simply need to get out there and move your body for at least three to six hours each week (thirty to sixty minutes per day, six days a week). But to give you some guidance on this issue, this chapter offers suggestions for "Interval Training" and "FlexSkills." I encourage you to follow through on these Vigor Improvement Practices (VIPs).

I know that many people claim they are "too busy" to exercise. In fact, being "too busy" is the most common excuse for not exercising. If you buy into that excuse, you need to accept the fact that your biochemical balance will never reach optimal levels and your vigor will suffer—simple as that. So I invite you to take a minute to think about all the things on which you regularly spend thirty to sixty minutes each day—television, newspapers, Internet, etc.—and then ask yourself if investing that same amount of time in your health and in how you feel is worthwhile. If you commit to an exercise program, I promise that your investment will produce great rewards.

[vip] INTERVAL TRAINING PLAN

Because I know how difficult it can be to push back against the stresses you face in the twenty-first century, I have developed a set of exercise recommendations that are designed to deliver the most benefits within the shortest time commitment possible. The most effective way to use exercise to restore biochemical balance and improve your vigor is with a three-times-weekly regimen of interval training (either running or walking). I think everyone would agree that walking is a pretty simple exercise that you can easily incorporate into your daily schedule. It doesn't require any fancy or expensive equipment, and you can do it virtually anywhere. To get the most from your walking regimen, you'll want to make sure you have a pair of comfortable and supportive shoes as well as approval from your personal health-care provider that it is okay for you to engage in moderate to vigorous exercise. Walk outside and enjoy the sights and sounds of your own neighborhood or a local park when the weather is good. Or when it is rainy or snowy, walk around the mall. Many shopping malls have organized walking groups that meet before the stores open and the mall becomes crowded with shoppers. When you get comfortable with walking on a regular basis, you can change the route and vary the intensity (walking faster or slower and adding hills or flats). Walking can also be part of developing your "mental" fitness as much as it serves as your "physical" exercise, because it can allow you some time to "get away" and to de-stress while your mind (and your body) wanders.

The Interval Training Plan described below has been used successfully by many of my clients and readers:

◈ Interval Training Plan

After a five-minute warm-up, the exercise alternates between high- and low-intensity levels as follows:

- ◈ one minute high intensity/one minute low intensity
- ◈ two minutes high intensity/two minutes low intensity
- ◈ three minutes high intensity/three minutes low intensity
- ◈ two minutes high intensity/two minutes low intensity
- ◈ one minute high intensity/one minute low intensity

Note that the intensity levels will be relative to your individual fitness level. A general guideline is that "high" intensity is not an "all-out effort" but rather a level that gets you breathing hard enough that you have difficulty carrying on a conversation with your exercise buddy. The "low" intensity intervals are easy enough to allow full recovery before your next hard interval — and also easy enough for you to talk without getting out of breath.

These eighteen minutes of interval training are followed by five minutes of easy cool-down exercise for a total duration of just under thirty minutes (twenty-eight minutes, to be exact). Compared to exercising at a steady/moderate "fat-burning" pace for this same twenty-eight minutes, the interval approach will burn more than double the number of calories (401 versus 189) and will result in superior biochemical balance via direct control of cortisol, testosterone, glucose, and other aspects of your biochemistry.

Exercise is a vital part of achieving and maintaining healthy biochemical balance and proper tissue repair. Whether we talk about joints, bones, muscles, tendons, or any other tissue, the right amount of the right type of exercise can help stimulate production of new collagen, removal of damaged tissue, and delivery of vital oxygen and nutrients. The body is designed to move. One famous philosopher commented that the human body is the only machine that breaks down from *underuse* rather than from overuse. (However, your body can break down from overuse as well, as evidenced by the numerous overtrained athletes that I have worked with over the years.) In many ways, the *motion* of exercise or any type of physical activity can be thought of as *lotion* for your joints and other tissues. The simple act of moving your body helps hydrate joints and stimulate tissue repair throughout the body, while the act of sitting around like a couch potato sends a constant "breakdown" signal (also called "atrophy") to your joint cartilage, bones, muscles, tendons, and ligaments.

[vip] FLEXSKILLS

In addition to the twenty-eight-minute walking program outlined above, you should consider also adding the flexibility exercises described below to further improve your circulation, balance, and strength. I call each of these ten exercises "FlexSkills," and I've used them to help elite athletes in virtually every type of sport improve their stress resilience, flexibility, and resistance to injury.

For each FlexSkill, you want to "hold" the position for thirty to sixty seconds. Each "cycle" of ten exercises, then, takes only five to ten minutes and can be performed either as a warm-up/cooldown on the days that you also do your Interval Walking or as an exercise circuit on its own. For example, you could go through all ten FlexSkills two or three times as your workout instead of walking. You may also want to use a floor mat or large towel when performing these skills.

◈ 1. Child's Pose (Targets: spine, lower back, shoulders, hips, knees, ankles)

This is one of the classic yoga poses — a resting and starting pose that serves as the base from which many other poses and stretches emanate. We'll use it as the initial FlexSkill, because it helps awaken and stimulate each of the major joint systems that we'll target with the subsequent FlexSkill movements.

From a standing position, come to your hands and knees. Point your toes so the tops of your feet are flat on the floor and your butt rests on your heels. Place your hands flat on the mat, about shoulders' width apart. Slowly reach forward, extending your arms straight out in front of you. Bend and extend your back and try to get your forehead as close to the floor as is comfortable. When you reach your farthest comfortable point, breath slowly and deeply, and hold this position for thirty to sixty seconds.

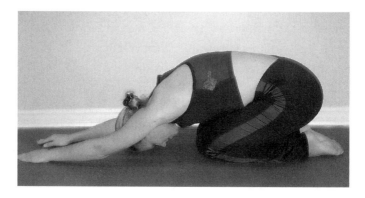

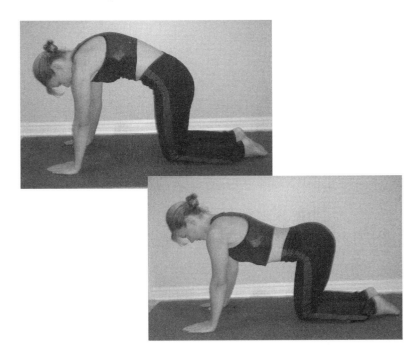

❖ 2. Arch (Targets: spine, neck, lower back, hips, abdominal
   area)

This FlexSkill is sometimes called "the Cat" by yoga instructors,
and it resembles a modified version of a standard yoga pose known
as "Downward-Facing Dog." You can move directly into the Arch
position from Child's Pose, or you can pause, take a breath, and
start from the kneeling position below.

From a "hand and knees" kneeling position, keep your hands
shoulders' width apart (directly beneath your shoulders). Slowly
arch your back upward (as a scared cat might arch its back) and
point your head downward using a count of five, pausing for another count of five at your highest arch point. Slowly arch your
back downward and your head upward, using the same five-sec-
ond count, pausing at your lowest arch point for another count of
five. Continue breathing deeply through three full repetitions of
arching upward and then downward for a total duration of sixty
seconds.

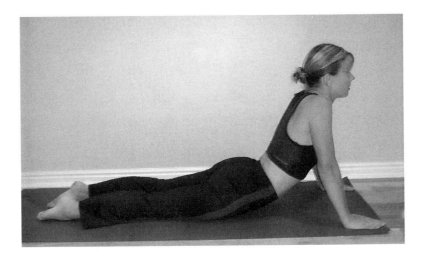

◈ 3. Cobra (Targets: spinal discs, lower back, front torso, hips, arms, and shoulders)

This position is also sometimes called "the Lizard" and has similarities to "the Upward-Facing Dog" pose in traditional yoga practice. Aside from the obvious advantage to your lower-back flexibility and spinal-disc alignment, the Cobra movement serves to open up and expand your entire front torso, an effect that will greatly improve your ability to breathe and thus to deliver vital oxygen to the repair process in every tissue.

Lying face down on your mat, place the palms of your hands under your shoulders. Inhale slowly and deeply, hold for a moment, and then, while slowly exhaling, push upward from your hands — raising your head and shoulders and allowing your lower back to naturally arch. Arch up as high as comfort allows, continue breathing slowly and deeply, and hold for thirty to sixty seconds. Slowly return to your beginning face-down lying position. As you become better at the Cobra FlexSkill, you will find it easier to push yourself into a fuller arch; for a more advanced movement, try arching your neck back to look toward the ceiling.

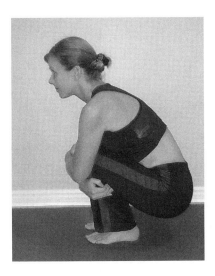

◈ 4. Squat (Targets: lower back, pelvis, hips, knees, ankles)

Okay, it is time to teach your skeleton what proper alignment looks like. This squat position is actually the "resting" position that is most natural in terms of skeletal alignment. Sitting in a chair (as most of us do for hours on end every day) is one of the worst biomechanical positions because of the extreme pressures, torques, and twists that the sitting position delivers to the back — especially to the lower back. Low-back pain affects eight out of ten American adults at some point in their lives, and the Squat helps realign the entire joint system into a more natural position.

Start in a standing position with your feet about shoulders' width apart and your toes pointing straight ahead. Take a deep breath and slowly squat down, bringing your butt to your ankles. Your hands can hang by your sides, or you can wrap them around your knees or position them on the ground in front or to the side of you to help balance yourself. Continue to breathe slowly and deeply, and hold the Squat position for thirty to sixty seconds. As your balance improves in the Squat position, you will find that you can maintain this comfortable position for many minutes without using your hands for balance or support.

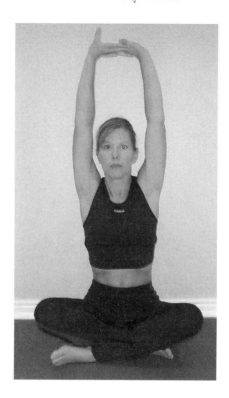

◈ 5. Sky Reach (Targets: spine and shoulders)

Also known as the "Pillar Stretch" and the "Mountain Pose" in yoga, this FlexSkill movement can be done seated or standing. I prefer to do the Sky Reach seated with my legs crossed, because I feel that I get a better low-back stretch in the seated position, and the next FlexSkill movement is also done in a seated position. But the choice is yours, and you may wish to experiment with seated and standing positions to see which you prefer.

From a cross-legged seated position (or standing with feet shoulders' width apart and toes pointing straight ahead), inhale slowly and deeply. Interlace your fingers, turn your palms away from your body, and reach for the sky. Look straight ahead, hold your spine straight, and breathe slowly and deeply. Hold your most comfortably extended position for thirty to sixty seconds.

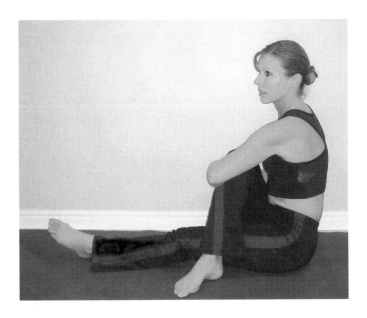

◈ 6. Figure-8 (Targets: lower back and hips)

Also called "the Pretzel" and "the Seated Hip Twist" in some forms of yoga, the Figure-8 FlexSkill is one of my personal favorites. As a runner and cyclist, my hips and lower back are in a constant state of stress, so this movement is vital to maintaining optimal flexibility and mobility in these important "core" areas.

From a seated position, with your legs straight out in front of you, keep your right leg straight and cross your left foot over to the outside of your right knee. Grasp the outside of your left knee and gently pull it toward the ribs on your right side. Slowly pull and continue breathing slowly and deeply until you feel a stretch in your left hip, butt, and lower back. Hold for twenty to thirty seconds. Slowly release the stretch, extend your left leg, and repeat the movement on your right knee.

◈ 7. Cross Twist (Targets: lower back, hips, spine, abdominal muscles)

This FlexSkill is a two-part movement, starting with a very simple "knee-to-chest" movement that you may have performed as a child in gym class, followed by the twisting position that is sometimes called a "T-Roll" or a "Crucifix Twist" because of the position of your upper body and arms during the movement.

Lying on your back with both legs out straight, use both hands to bring your right knee up to your chest. Take a deep breath, and with your hands on your knee/shin, slowly pull your right leg/knee into your chest until you can feel a gentle stretch in your lower back and right hip. Pull as far as you feel comfortable, and hold for fifteen to thirty seconds while you continue to breathe slowly and deeply.

At the end of your "hold," slowly extend your hands outward to your sides, forming a "T" shape with your body. Slowly rotate your pelvis and torso to lower your right knee toward your left side, bringing the inside of your right knee as close to your mat as possible while keeping your palms and shoulders flat on your mat. At your most comfortable twist position, continue to breathe slowly and deeply, and hold for fifteen to thirty seconds. Repeat both positions (knee-to-chest and twist) with your left leg.

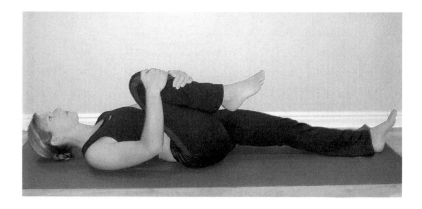

As you become more flexible and can pull your leg/knee farther into your chest and rotate your knee closer to touching your mat, you may also begin to feel a gentle stretch in your opposite hip flexor (the front part of your hip — an area that becomes very tight in many people and causes extreme strain to lower-back muscles).

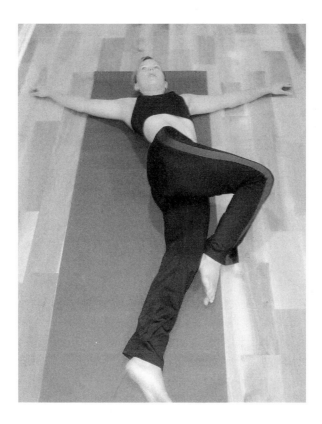

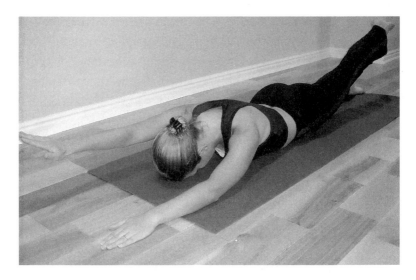

◆ 8. Superman (Targets: lower back, spine, hips, shoulders, neck, and shoulders)

Also known as "the Locust" position in some forms of yoga, the Superman position is popular as much for its strengthening and balancing qualities as for its flexibility benefits. As a FlexSkill, the Superman movement can be performed in several variations, from easy to advanced, depending on your degree of flexibility.

Start from a lying face-down position, with your forehead flat on your mat. Your arms should be stretched out in front of you with your palms flat on the floor. Breathe slowly and deeply for a few moments. Keeping your forehead flat on the mat, slowly raise your *right* hand/arm and *left* foot/leg off the mat as far as comfort allows. You should feel a slight stretch in your front torso and through your entire back, hip, and butt region. *If you feel any low-back pain at all, you should lower your hand and/or foot until you feel comfortable again.* Continue taking slow/deep breaths, and hold this extended position for fifteen to thirty seconds. Slowly lower your right hand and left foot, take a deep breath in the beginning (face-down) position, and repeat the movement with your left hand and right foot.

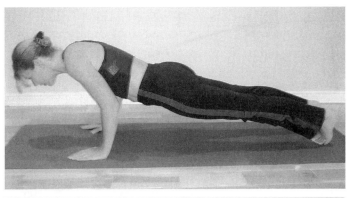

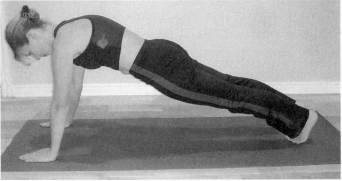

◈ 9. Plank (Targets: spine, upper/lower back muscles, hips, abdominal muscles ankles, shoulders, arms)

This movement is a classic yoga position that helps integrate upper and lower body alignment. You can think of the Plank as a static "push-up" in high and low positions. Start this FlexSkill with the "high" position and progress to the "low" position. In doing so, you encourage muscle activity in all parts of the body and stimulate circulation and delivery of nutrients to a range of connective tissues. Breathing is an important consideration in this FlexSkill, because, with so many muscles being activated, you'll have to concentrate on taking full, deep breaths for the entire movement.

Start from the same relaxed face-down position as the Superman movement (#8 on the previous page). Place your hands, palms down, directly under your shoulders. Take a deep, cleansing breath, and fully extend your arms, pushing upward to the "high" Plank position. Try to stay up on your toes while you maintain a straight spine and neck, and focus your eyes on the floor directly in front of your fingertips. Concentrate on maintaining slow, deep, even breaths, and hold this position for fifteen to thirty seconds. This can be a very challenging movement, especially if you lack a lot of upper-body strength, so only maintain this "high" position for as long as you feel comfortable. You will then move directly into the "low" Plank position by simply allowing your arms to slowly bend and bringing your elbows to the side of your body. Continuing to breathe slowly and deeply, hold this position for fifteen to thirty seconds before slowly returning to your face-down starting position with your stomach flat on your mat. Take another deep, cleansing breath.

◈ 10. Multi-Split (Targets: spine, upper/lower back, hips, abdominal muscles, legs, ankles, shoulders, and arms)

This FlexSkill is another two-part movement that targets multiple joints simultaneously, while at the same time improving muscle strength and balance. The primary idea behind this movement is to get the upper- and lower-body connective tissues aligned and working in concert with one another. In some forms of yoga, this Multi-Split movement is known as "the Stork" or "the Tree" and sometimes as the "Crescent Lunge," depending on the direction of the movement.

Start from a standing position with your toes pointing straight ahead and your arms at your sides. Take a deep, cleansing breath. In the first part of the movement, extend your arms upward and away from your sides so they are parallel to the floor. Then, bring the sole of your right foot slowly up the inside of your left leg, raising your right foot as high as feels comfortable for you. Continue maintaining a slow, deep rhythmic breathing pattern (and your balance!) as you hold this position for fifteen to thirty seconds.

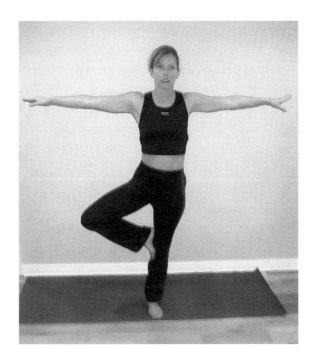

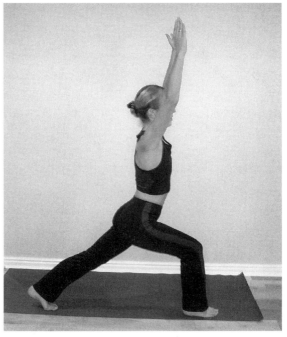

Slowly return your right foot to your mat and repeat on the other side.

In the second part of this FlexSkill, you will start from the same standing/toes-forward/arms-at-side position. Take a deep, cleansing breath, look straight ahead, and step forward with your right foot. Keeping both knees pointing straight ahead, bend your right knee into as deep a lunge as feels comfortable. Continue your slow, deep breathing while you reach your arms upward straight over your head. Imagine lengthening your spine from your lower back all the way up to the ceiling with each breath. Hold this position for fifteen to thirty seconds before slowly returning your arms to your sides and stepping back from your lunge into your starting position. Repeat with your left leg.

After finishing this last FlexSkill movement, you should come back to a resting position for a few last deep, cleansing breaths. You can use a comfortable standing position, the Squat position, or even the Child's Pose to bring it all together to a relaxing conclusion. Experiment with each position to determine how you best like to end each FlexSkill session, or try ending with a different position each time.

10

[vigor improvement practices]

Dietary Supplements

Natural dietary supplements are known to effectively and safely influence the stress response and can help restore biochemical balance in each of the Four Pillars of Health. In this chapter, each supplement is described in terms of the scientific and medical evidence for its effects on vigor. Recommendations for safety, dosage levels, and what to look for if you decide to use the supplement are also provided.

Dietary supplements, including vitamins, minerals, herbs/extracts, and amino acids are extremely safe. As the author of two academic textbooks on the subject of dietary supplements, I believe it is worth noting that when supplements are used as directed, any adverse events or side effects are exceedingly rare. That said, they do happen from time to time, and they are almost impossible to predict because of differences between product formulations, individual health statuses, medication regimens, and numerous lifestyle factors (diet, sleep, stress, etc.). For example, any individual who is under medical supervision for a chronic disease or who is taking prescription or over-the-counter medications should always check with their health-care provider before adding any dietary supplement to their daily regimen. Likewise, women should understand that any dietary supplement that they are considering taking is unlikely to have been researched or found to be safe under conditions of pregnancy or lactation, so it is best to avoid these supplements during these high-risk times of life.

WHY TAKE SUPPLEMENTS?

Because so many strategies for reducing stress and increasing vigor are available, some people question whether they really need nutritional supplements. But I counter by asking them, "Why *not* take supplements?" In research and in real life, I have seen the value of a strategic regimen of carefully chosen natural dietary supplements. These supplements can help restore biochemical balance within and between each of the Four Pillars of Health: manage oxidation, control inflammation, stabilize glucose, and balance stress hormones.

Let's admit it: For most people, from a purely practical perspective, developing a regimen for biochemical balance that incorporates appropriate dietary supplementation is usually more "doable" than following a complicated stress-management program or making time for regular exercise. This does not at all imply that stress management is unimportant or that supplements can provide all the same benefits that exercise delivers. Nevertheless, supplements, for many people, represent a habit that they can incorporate into their already-busy daily lives, and supplements can have powerfully beneficial effects on controlling stress and restoring vigor.

Whether your exposure to stress is the result of physical or psychological factors, the response mounted by the body's hormonal system is exactly the same and just as detrimental. This means physical stressors, such as suboptimal nutrition (dieting), extremes of exercise (too much or too little), inadequate sleep, or even "aging," will affect the body in many of the same ways as psychological stressors, such as concerns about bills, traffic, deadlines, family worries, etc. No matter what source of stress a person is exposed to, the body proceeds through a systemic stress response that eventually leads to problems with biochemical balance, reduced vigor, and declining health. However, advances in nutritional science and biochemistry have shown that a wide variety of dietary and herbal ingredients can assist the body in mounting an adaptive response to stress and help minimize or control some of the systemic detrimental health effects of stress.

These natural products represent a logical and convenient approach for many people who are subjected to stressors on a daily basis — for example, from work, finances, or the environment. Most of the time, "removing" the stressor (avoiding it) is an impossible option, no matter how desirable that option may be. Think about it: You have to work (stress!), you have to pay your bills on time (stress!), you may have to sit in rush-hour traffic (stress!), and you have family and interpersonal relationships that don't always go smoothly (stress!). You also know that you should be "eating better" and that you should be "getting more exercise" (both of which can help control the stress response), but the reality of your busy life means that other things often take priority over exercise — jobs, kids, spouses, chores…you name it. In addition, the very concept of taking time out of your busy schedules for a yoga or meditation class may be downright laughable, even though you know it would likely do you a lot of good.

For some people, a properly formulated supplement regimen may be the "last piece of the puzzle" that helps them finally restore biochemical balance in their bodies. For others, the supplements may be the "first step" toward getting their metabolism back on an even keel and allowing them to incorporate other healthy lifestyle choices, such as regular exercise and proper diet. For many people, the only logical solution to managing an overactive stress response and restoring vigor may be the use of targeted dietary supplements to help establish and maintain the body's biochemical balance.

VITAMINS AND VIGOR

It almost goes without saying that taking a general multivitamin and mineral supplement is a good idea for anybody who is under stress, maintains a hectic lifestyle, or needs more vigor. Every energy-related reaction that takes place in the body, especially those involved in the stress response, relies in one way or another on vitamins and minerals as "cofactors" to make the reactions go. For example, B-complex vitamins are needed for metabolism of protein and carbohydrate, chromium is involved in handling carbohydrates, magnesium and calcium are needed for proper muscle contraction, zinc and copper are required as enzyme cofactors in nearly three hundred separate reactions, iron is needed to help shuttle oxygen in the blood — the list goes on and on.

It is fairly well accepted in the medical community that subclinical or marginal deficiencies of essential micronutrients, especially the B vitamins and magnesium, can lead to psychological and physiological symptoms that are related to stress. Many studies show that various combinations of vitamins and minerals reduce oxidation and inflammation, help control blood sugar, improve immune-system function, and generally improve overall health and well-being. Surveys show that "most" health professionals take daily multivitamins, and scientific evidence generally supports the rationale behind using a general nutritional supplement as a foundation on which to build a solid regimen of biochemical balance.

DIETARY SUPPLEMENTS AND
THE FOUR PILLARS OF HEALTH

Rather than write another encyclopedia about dietary supplements, I want to use this chapter to give you a somewhat brief, but hopefully practical, overview of some of the vitamins and nutritional supplements that I have found over the years to be most beneficial for restoring biochemical balance in the Four Pillars of Health. If you want more details for each supplement, I invite you to see the Resources section of this book for some recommended textbooks specializing in dietary supplement science, including the traditional use, scientific evidence, safety, and dosing recommendations for a wide range of potentially beneficial dietary supplements.

Even though a great deal of the biochemistry presented in earlier sections may appear to be a bit complicated and overwhelming, the overall picture is really quite simple. You basically want to *stop* excessive levels of oxidation, inflammation, glycation, and stress-hormone exposure. By reining in these destructive biochemical forces, you can slow the breakdown of your tissues and enhance their restoration. At the same time, you want to *enhance* the process of repair and rebuilding of those damaged tissues — and restoring biochemical balance allows the body to do its job of repair much faster and more completely. Finally, you also want to *protect* the new healthy tissue from future damage by maintaining your biochemical balance and keeping it from becoming unbalanced again. If your biochemistry is balanced and your tissues are functioning optimally, then you'll "feel" that balance in terms of a high perception of vigor. Remember, as stated in the beginning of this book: "Balance your biochemistry to beat burnout!"

You've already been introduced to the idea that it is important to take a simple daily multivitamin containing B-complex vitamins, vitamins C and D, and such minerals as calcium and magnesium. The forthcoming sections discuss what roles specific vitamins can play in strengthening the Four Pillars of Health. I also provide you with information on a targeted blend of herbs for restoring biochemical balance, such as eurycoma, citrus PMFs (polymethoxylated flavones), green-tea catechins, theanine, and others.

To make it easier for you to see the link between dietary supplements and specific pathways to greater vigor, I have broken down the rest of the chapter into sections that address each of the Four Pillars of Health.

[vip] SUPPLEMENTS FOR MANAGING OXIDATION

Antioxidant nutrients are important for controlling the activity of the highly reactive oxygen molecules known as free radicals, because unchecked free-radical activity is what leads to the cellular damage known as "oxidation" and the cycle of glycation and inflammation that follows, causing additional damage and dysfunction. As mentioned earlier when I discussed the "Antioxidant Network," remember it is the overall *collection* and *balance* of several antioxidants that is important rather than any single "super" antioxidant. Your cells need representatives of all five major classes of antioxidants to mount the strongest antioxidant defenses: vitamin-E complex, vitamin-C complex, thiols, carotenoids, and flavonoids.

◈ Vitamin C

Vitamin C, also known as ascorbic acid, is a water-soluble vitamin needed by the body for hundreds of vital metabolic reactions. Good food sources of vitamin C include all citrus fruits (oranges, grapefruit, lemons), as well as many other fruits and vegetables, such as strawberries, tomatoes, broccoli, brussels sprouts, peppers, and cantaloupe.

Perhaps the most well-known function of vitamin C is as one of the key nutritional antioxidants, where it protects the body from free-radical damage. As a water-soluble vitamin, ascorbic acid performs its antioxidant functions within the aqueous compartments of the blood and inside cells and can help restore the antioxidant potential of vitamin E (a fat-soluble antioxidant).

Although the recommended daily allowance (RDA) for vitamin C has recently been raised from 60 mg to 75 to 90 mg (higher for men), it is well established that almost everybody can benefit from higher levels. For example, the vitamin C recommendation for cigarette smokers is 100 to 200 mg per day, because smoking destroys vitamin C in the body. Full blood and tissue saturation is achieved with daily intakes of 200 to 500 mg per day, and the absorption and activity of vitamin C (ascorbic acid) is approximately tripled when supplemented in combination with flavonoids.

◈ Vitamin E

Vitamin E is actually a family of related compounds known as tocopherols and tocotrienols. Although alpha-tocopherol is the most common form found in dietary supplements, vitamin E also exists with slightly different chemical structures, such as beta-, gamma-, and delta-tocopherol as well as alpha-, beta-, gamma-, and delta-tocotrienols — and natural forms of all eight structures are important for overall health.

Vitamin E can be obtained as a supplement in natural or synthetic form. In most cases, the natural and synthetic form of vitamins and minerals are identical, but in the case of vitamin E, the natural form ("d-") is clearly superior in terms of absorption and retention in the body compared to its synthetic ("dl-") counterpart (about double compared to synthetic forms).

◈ Beta-carotene

Beta-carotene is part of a large family of compounds known as carotenoids (which includes more than six hundred members, such as lycopene and lutein). Carotenoids are widely distributed in fruits and vegetables and are responsible, along with flavonoids, for contributing the color to many plants (a rule of thumb is the brighter, the better). In terms of nutrition, beta-carotene's primary role is as a precursor to vitamin A (the body can convert beta-carotene into vitamin A as it is needed). It is important to note that beta-carotene and vitamin A are often described in the same breath, almost as if they were the same compound (which they are not). Although beta-carotene can be converted to vitamin A in the body, important differences in terms of action and safety exist between the two compounds. Beta-carotene, like most carotenoids, is also a powerful antioxidant and is especially effective at preventing inflammatory damage. The best food sources are brightly colored fruits and veggies, such as cantaloupe, apricots, carrots, red peppers, sweet potatoes, and dark, leafy greens.

◈ Green Tea

Green tea (*Camellia sinensis*) is the second most consumed beverage in the world (water is the first), and it has been used medicinally for centuries in India and China. The active constituents in green tea are a family of polyphenols (catechins) with antioxidant activity about twenty-five to one hundred times more potent than vitamins C and E. A cup of green tea may provide 10 to 40 mg of polyphenols and has antioxidant activity greater than a serving of broccoli, spinach, carrots, or strawberries. Because the active compounds (the catechins) found in green tea are known to possess potent antioxidant activity, they may provide beneficial health effects by protecting the body from the damaging effects of oxidative damage from free radicals. From laboratory findings, it is clear that green tea is an effective antioxidant, that it provides clear protection from experimentally induced DNA damage, and that it can slow or halt the initiation and progression of oxidation and inflammation. Several epidemiological studies show an association between consumption of total flavonoids in the diet and the risk for inflammatory conditions. Men with the highest consumption of flavonoids (from fruits and vegetables) have approximately half the risk of heart disease and cancer (both are oxidative and inflammatory diseases) compared with those with the lowest intake.

◈ Beta-glucan

Beta-glucan is a generic term for "beta-1,3-linked polyglucose," which is a polysaccharide (basically a long chain of sugar molecules) found in the cell walls of yeast cells and some plants. Purified beta-glucan (derived from yeast) is known to help the immune system better fight off infections, cold/flu viruses, and cancer/tumors. When out of balance (high or low), the immune system not only fails to protect the body from invading pathogens (bacteria and viruses) but can even attack it, mistaking the body's own cells for dangerous pathogens, resulting in oxidative and inflammatory autoimmune diseases, such as lupus and rheumatoid arthritis. Allergies can result when the immune system is "overactive" and mistakes an innocuous and harmless particle (such as pollen or cat dander) for an invading pathogen. Another side effect of an immune system that is out of balance is chronic low-grade inflammation, which can increase risks for cancer and heart disease and other chronic diseases related to elevated inflammation. By controlling and "guiding" the activity of the innate immune system, beta-glucan supplements can help modulate systemic levels of oxidation/inflammation in the body and thus help maintain biochemical balance and improve vigor.

[vip] SUPPLEMENTS FOR CONTROLLING INFLAMMATION

Recall from earlier sections that the general idea with inflammation is that you want "enough" — not too much and not too little — but that balance can become upset by poor diet, disease, injury, stress, and other lifestyle factors. Some researchers would go so far as to say that "overinflammation" is at the heart of virtually every disease process, including burnout or low vigor, and certainly the data support a strong link between inflammation and heart disease, cancer, obesity, and Alzheimer's disease (not to mention the long list of clearly "inflammatory" diseases, such as fibromyalgia, rheumatoid arthritis, lupus, and others). Other sections of this book cover some of the most effective natural approaches for keeping inflammation under control, including reducing your intake of refined carbohydrates, increasing your intake of omega-3 fatty acids and brightly colored fruits and vegetables, as well as reducing stress-hormone exposure. The information that follows outlines some of the most effective dietary supplements for naturally controlling inflammation.

◈ Mangosteen

One of my favorite natural supplements for controlling inflammation is mangosteen (*Garcinia mangostana*), the fruit of a family of trees and shrubs that grow in tropical climates, especially in Asia, Polynesia, and South Africa. Mangosteen fruit is often called the "Queen of Fruits" due to its pleasant flavor and its widespread use in traditional medicine. The mangosteen fruit is round, with a smooth, thick, firm rind that is pale green when immature and dark purple or red-purple when ripe. Enclosed by the rind are four to eight white segments of edible pulp. The mangosteen fruit contains a family of anti-inflammatory and antioxidant compounds called xanthones. The plant is also a rich source of other bioactive molecules, including flavonoids, benzophenones, lactones, and phenolic acids. Mangosteen fruit preparations (typically "puréed" concoctions that include the fruit and the rind, or pericarp, where the majority of the bioactive xanthones are concentrated) have been used for antioxidant protection against free radicals, promoting joint flexibility, reducing joint inflammation, and preventing cancer — but one of the most effective uses of whole-fruit mangosteen puree is to control inflammation and restore overall biochemical balance, because it simultaneously controls oxidation and inflammation.

◈ Essential Fatty Acids

The term "essential fatty acids" refers to two fatty acids — linoleic acid and linolenic acid — that the body cannot synthesize and thus must be consumed in the diet (vitamins and minerals are also termed "essential," because the body cannot make them and therefore must consume them). These essential fatty acids are needed for the production of compounds known as cytokines, which help regulate inflammation, blood clotting, blood pressure, heart rate, immune response, and a wide variety of other biological processes.

Linoleic acid is considered an "omega-6" (n-6) fatty acid. It is found in vegetable and nut oils, such as sunflower, safflower, corn, soy, and peanut oil. Most Americans get adequate levels of these omega-6 oils in their diets, due to a high consumption of vegetable oil–based margarine and salad dressings. Linolenic acid is classified as an "omega-3" (n-3) fatty acid. Good dietary sources are flaxseed oil (51 percent linolenic acid), soy oil (7 percent), walnuts (7 percent), and canola oil (9 percent), as well as margarine derived from canola oil. For example, a tablespoon of canola oil or canola oil margarine provides about 1 g of linolenic acid.

If you think back to the type of diet humans evolved to eat (caveman diet), it provided a much more balanced mix of n-3 and n-6 fatty acids. Over the last century, modern diets have come to rely heavily on fats derived from vegetable oils (n-6), bringing the ratio of n-6 to n-3 fatty acids from the caveman's ratio of 1:1 to the modern-day range of 20:1 or 30:1! The unbalanced intake of high n-6 fatty acids and low n-3 fatty acids sets the stage for increases in various inflammatory processes.

Fatty acids of the n-3 variety have opposing biological effects to the n-6 fatty acids, meaning that a higher intake of n-3 oils can deliver anti-inflammatory, antithrombotic, and vasodilatory effects that can lead to benefits in terms of heart disease, hypertension, diabetes, and a wide variety of inflammatory conditions, such as fibromyalgia, rheumatoid arthritis, and ulcerative colitis.

In the body, linoleic acid (n-6) is metabolized into arachidonic acid, a precursor to specific "bad" cytokines that can promote vasoconstriction, elevated blood pressure, and painful inflammation. Linolenic acid (n-3) is metabolized in the body to EPA (eicosapentaenoic acid) and DHA (docosahexaenoic acid). EPA serves as the precursor to prostaglandin E3, which has anti-inflammatory properties that can counteract the inflammation caused by n-6 fatty acids.

Recent studies have shown that consumption of linolenic acid and other n-3 fatty acids offers wide-ranging anti-inflammatory benefits. This effect is thought to be mediated through the synthesis of EPA and DHA. Fish oils contain large amounts of EPA and DHA, and the majority of studies in this area have used various concentrations of fish-oil supplements to demonstrate the health benefits of these essential fatty acids. For example, 1 g of menhaden oil (a common fish used to produce fish-oil supplements) provides about 300 mg of these fatty acids. EPA is known to induce an anti-inflammatory effect through its inhibition of cyclooxygenase (which converts arachidonic acid to thromboxane A2).

Some evidence suggests that omega-3 fatty acids from fish oil and flaxseed may help improve insulin sensitivity (thus reducing glycation) and reduce perception of stress (thus reducing cortisol exposure). A recent expert scientific advisory board at the National Institutes of Health highlighted the importance of a balanced intake of n-6 and n-3 fatty acids to reduce the adverse effects of elevated (inflammatory) arachidonic acid (a metabolic product of n-6 metabolism). The committee recommended a reduction in the intake of n-6 fatty acids (linoleic acid) and an increase in n-3 (linolenic acid, DHA, EPA) intake.

No serious adverse side effects should be expected from regular consumption of essential fatty acid supplements, whether from fish oil or other common oil supplements (see below). However, due to the tendency of n-3 fatty acids to reduce platelet aggregation ("thin" the blood), increased bleeding times can occur in some individuals.

The best dietary sources of omega-3 fatty acids are fish, such as trout, tuna, salmon, mackerel, herring, and sardines, which all contain 1 to 2 g of n-3 oils per three- to four-ounce serving. A minimum of 4 to 5 g of linoleic acid (but no more than 6 to 7 g) and 2 to 3 g of linolenic acid are recommended per day. Supplements of linoleic acid (n-6) are typically not needed, whereas linolenic acid (n-3) supplements (4 to 10 g/d) or concentrated EPA/DHA supplements (400 to 1,000 mg/d) are recommended to balance normal inflammatory processes. Total DHA/EPA intake should approach about 1 g per day, evenly split between the two.

In addition to fish oils, other plant-derived oils are rich sources of essential fatty acids, including flaxseed, borage seed, and evening primrose.

◈ Evening Primrose Oil

Evening primrose oil (EPO) is most commonly used for relieving inflammatory conditions associated with "women's health," such as premenstrual syndrome, fibrocystic breasts, and menopausal symptoms, such as hot flashes. Each of these conditions is related on a biochemical level to an excessive inflammatory response.

The essential fatty acid linoleic acid forms 60 to 80 percent of evening primrose oil, but the gamma linoleic acid (GLA) component of EPO may be more important for controlling inflammation. The body synthesizes GLA from linoleic acid, which comprises 8 to 14 percent of the oil in EPO supplements. GLA is a precursor of prostaglandin E1 (PGE1), a deficiency of which has been documented in some women with premenstrual syndrome (PMS) and cyclical breast pain. Because decreased levels of PGE1 can increase the pain-inducing effect of the hormone prolactin on breast tissue, it is thought that they may be a primary cause of many of the symptoms associated with PMS.

PGE1 has beneficial anti-inflammatory effects, and supplementation with EPO is known to control a variety of inflammatory disorders. In a double-blind crossover study in men taking either fish oil alone or fish oil plus EPO, the combination lead to a significant 12 percent decrease in inflammatory markers, whereas fish oil alone lead to a 6 percent decrease in the same markers.

◈ Borage Oil

Borage seeds are a rich source of a GLA (20 to 30 percent of total oil content), which has medicinal properties that have been demonstrated in such areas as anti-inflammatory activity, immune-system modulation, management of atopic eczema (excessive proliferation of the skin cells), and other skin maladies. Studies have shown that individuals with active rheumatoid arthritis (an inflammatory condition) experienced an improvement in their symptoms when they were given a borage oil supplement daily for six months.

◈ Boswellia

The boswellia plant (*Boswellia serrata*) produces a sap that has been used in traditional Indian medicine as a treatment for arthritis and inflammatory conditions. The primary compounds thought to be responsible for the anti-inflammatory activity of boswellia are known as boswellic acids. These compounds are known to interfere with enzymes that contribute to inflammation and pain (COX-2, 5-LO, and 12-LO).

Boswellia sap/resin has a long history of safe and effective use as a mild anti-inflammatory to reduce pain and stiffness and promote increased mobility (without many of the associated gastrointestinal side effects commonly reported for synthetic anti-inflammatory medications). A number of studies have shown that boswellic acids may possess anti-inflammatory activity at least as potent as common over-the-counter medications, such as ibuprofen and aspirin. In one study of patients with rheumatoid arthritis, pain and swelling were reduced following three months of boswellia use. In some cases, boswellia may be associated with mild gastrointestinal upset (heartburn, aftertaste, and nausea — so take it with food), but no serious adverse side effects have been reported.

❖ Bromelain and Papain

The term "proteolytic" is a catch-all term referring to enzymes that digest protein. In the body, proteolytic enzymes, such as bromelain (from pineapples) and papain (from papayas), act as anti-inflammatory agents and pain relievers and have been effective in accelerating recovery from exercise and injury in athletes, as well as tissue repair in patients following surgery. In one study of soccer players suffering from ankle injuries, proteolytic-enzyme supplements accelerated healing and got players back on the field about 50 percent faster than athletes assigned to receive placebo tablets. A handful of other small trials in athletes have shown enzymes can help reduce inflammation, speed healing of bruises and other tissue injuries, and reduce overall recovery time when compared to athletes taking placebos.

❖ Flaxseed Oil

Flaxseed is just what it sounds like—the seed of the flax plant. Flaxseed is typically used as a source of the essential fatty acids linolenic acid (LN) and linoleic acid (LA). Flaxseed oil is about 57 percent LN (an omega-3) and about 17 percent LA (an omega-6). LN can be converted into EPA and DHA, fatty acids that are precursors to anti-inflammatory and anti-atherogenic prostaglandins.

Regular flaxseed consumption has been associated with improvements in the ratio of omega-3 to omega-6 fatty acids in the blood, a situation that may offer protection and relief from inflammatory conditions. A number of animal and human studies on flaxseed oil have shown a clear and consistent reduction in pro-inflammatory markers (tumor-necrosis factor and interleukins).

❖ Ginger

Ginger (*Zingiber officinale*) has been used throughout history as an aid for many gastrointestinal disturbances, as well as for relief of inflamed joints. The most active chemical compounds in ginger are known as the gingerols, which are also the most aromatic compounds in this root and are thought to be the reason that ginger can inhibit substances that cause the pain and inflammation associated with osteoarthritis. For example, in osteoarthritis patients taking powdered ginger, 75 percent of the subjects reported decreased pain and swelling after treatment with ginger for one month. Ginger supplementation is known to reduce production of the inflammatory thromboxane compounds associated with excess inflammation and pain. In studies of patients with osteoarthritis and rheumatoid arthritis, significant pain relief was noted in more than half (55 percent) of the osteoarthritis patients and nearly three-quarters (74 percent) of the rheumatoid arthritis patients when supplemented with ginger.

◈ Turmeric

Turmeric is known by the Latin plant name *Curcuma longa* (where the name for the turmeric-derived spice "curcumin" comes from) and is a member of the ginger family (Zingiberaceae). As a traditional medicine, turmeric is used as an anti-inflammatory, antioxidant, and analgesic (pain reliever). Currently, research is continuing to investigate turmeric's anti-inflammatory effects and its potential as a potent anticancer agent (which makes sense if cancer is viewed as an inflammatory disease). The primary active compounds in turmeric are the flavonoid curcumin and related "curcuminoid" compounds that deliver potent antioxidant, anti-inflammatory, and chemoprotective (anticancer) effects. As such, turmeric-containing supplements would logically be expected to have a beneficial effect in such areas as arthritis, cancer, and heart disease. In a wide range of animal studies, turmeric extracts have been shown to significantly alleviate the pain of arthritis (naturally occurring and experimentally induced forms). In human studies, arthritis pain and a variety of inflammatory compounds, including cyclooxygenase-2 (COX-2) and 5-lipoxygenase (5-LO), were controlled by turmeric. In a particular series of experiments at

Houston's MD Anderson Cancer Center, turmeric extracts have been shown to control the inflammatory cascade associated with a variety of inflammatory diseases, including cancer, atherosclerosis, arthritis, and osteoporosis.

❖ Vitamin D

You probably think of vitamin D as being "good for strong bones" and helping prevent osteoporosis — and that is true, because it helps the body absorb calcium from the diet. The more recent and exciting news is that vitamin D can help reduce the risk of a wide range of diseases, including diabetes, heart attacks, high blood pressure, chronic pain, multiple sclerosis, depression, stroke, rheumatoid arthritis, and cancers of the lung, prostate, kidney, esophagus, breast, ovary, stomach, and bladder. Vitamin D also acts as an immune-system modulator, preventing excessive expression of inflammatory cytokines and increasing the "oxidative-burst" potential of macrophages.

Scientific evidence also suggests that vitamin-D deficiency is responsible for immune-related conditions, including autism and asthma. For example, the seasonal vitamin-D deficiency that spikes during the winter months (when sun exposure is reduced) has been associated with immune-system dysfunction, including autoimmune disease, such as multiple sclerosis (MS), type 1 diabetes, rheumatoid arthritis, and autoimmune thyroid disease. Many scientists have even suggested that the vitamin-D deficiency that comes with the winter months may be the seasonal trigger for influenza outbreaks around the world.

Very few foods are good sources of vitamin D, and they include fortified dairy products and breakfast cereals, fatty fish, beef liver (which is too high in vitamin A), and egg yolks. Cod-liver oil is a good source of vitamin D but also tends to contain too much vitamin A, which can interfere with the absorption and activity of vitamin D in the body. The two forms of vitamin D found in dietary supplements are D-2 (ergocalciferol) and D-3 (cholecalciferol), with D-3 being the preferred form, because it is chemically equal to the form of vitamin D produced by the body and is two to three times more effective than the D-2 form at raising blood levels of vitamin D. A daily dose of 2,000 IU of vitamin D-3 would be expected to raise blood levels by 20 ng/mL, which is about the amount of "deficiency" that the average person might expect to have (especially during the winter months in a northern-latitude city in the United States).

[vip] SUPPLEMENTS FOR STABILIZING GLUCOSE

When most people think of controlling blood sugar, they automatically think about diabetes (which affects about twenty-five million Americans, with 90 to 95 percent of cases manifesting as "Type II" diabetes). At least double that number — more than fifty million Americans — have what might be called "prediabetes," or a dysfunctional or suboptimal control of blood sugar. Most of these people are completely unaware that their blood-sugar levels are fluctuating wildly throughout the day, but they clearly feel the effects in terms of fatigue, problems concentrating, constant hunger, weight gain, and accelerated aging — mostly via glycation, but also via oxidation and inflammation.

Optimal control of blood sugar — and the excessive glycation that can result from improper control — can be greatly enhanced by consuming a number of the dietary supplements outlined below.

◈ Licorice Root

Licorice root *(Glycyrrhiza glabra)* has been used by practitioners of traditional medicine around the world for at least four thousand years — especially in Egyptian and Middle-Eastern medicine, where licorice plants are thought to have originated. Licorice roots contain bioactive polyphenols, predominantly glabridin, which possess antioxidant, glucose-lowering, anti-inflammatory, and antistress properties. Perhaps the most beneficial effect of licorice/glabridin extracts is their ability to reduce abdominal fat and blood glucose in diabetic or overweight subjects. In one six-week study of moderately overweight men and women, a once-daily glabridin supplement reduced glucose levels by 10 percent, controlled appetite, and induced a one-pound per week loss of body fat, with no significant alterations to diet or exercise patterns.

◈ Alpha-Lipoic Acid

Alpha-lipoic acid has been established by many European and U.S. studies as an important antioxidant *and* blood-sugar controller. Alpha-lipoic acid has been named "the universal antioxidant," because it reacts with many different free radicals. Alpha-lipoic acid supplementation enhances insulin action and can reduce or reverse oxidative nerve damage caused by elevated blood-sugar levels. In conjunction with other antioxidants, such as vitamin E, alpha-lipoic acid may be doubly helpful in patients with diabetes. By promoting the production of energy from fat and sugar in the mitochondria, glucose removal from the bloodstream may be enhanced and insulin function improved. Indeed, alpha-lipoic acid has been shown to decrease insulin resistance and is prescribed frequently in Europe as a treatment for peripheral neuropathy (nerve damage) associated with diabetes. In the United States, the American Diabetes Association has suggested that alpha-lipoic acid plus vitamin E may be helpful in combating some of the health complications associated with diabetes, including heart disease, vision problems, nerve damage, and kidney disease.

◈ Chromium

Chromium is a trace mineral that is essential for normal insulin function, but dietary studies indicate that most people in the United States and other industrialized countries simply don't get enough chromium, and deficiencies appear to be even more common in people with diabetes and problems with blood-sugar control. Chromium also aids in the metabolism of glucose, regulation of insulin levels, and maintenance of healthy blood levels of cholesterol and other lipids. Chromium forms part of a compound in the body known as glucose tolerance factor (GTF), which is involved in regulating the actions of insulin in maintaining blood-sugar levels and, possibly, in helping control appetite. Food sources include brewer's yeast, whole-grain cereals, broccoli, prunes, mushrooms, and beer. (Note: Most of the calories in beer come from the alcohol — about 100–150 calories of the total 150–200 calories in a 12 oz beer — while carbs only account for 40–80 calories, depending on the brand of beer. I'm not advocating that diabetics start gulping beer to get their chromium, but beer is one of the "foods" that delivers a decent supply of chromium into the food supply.) Many clinical studies support the benefits and safety of chromium supplementation for normalizing blood sugar. Supplemental chromium can lower blood-insulin levels, improve glucose tolerance, and decrease systemic levels of glycation. Experts from the U.S. Department of Agriculture at the Beltsville Human Nutrition Research Center recommend chromium supplementation in daily amounts of 200 mcg for optimal blood-sugar control.

◈ Fenugreek

Fenugreek is a well-known spice that has been used in Asia and Africa to treat various ailments, including diabetes. The active, blood-sugar lowering principles of fenugreek have not been entirely elucidated, but dietary fiber and saponins (which are also antioxidants) may contribute. Fenugreek seeds contain an amino acid (4-hydroxyisoleucine) that may stimulate insulin secretion (direct beta-cell stimulation) and help control blood-sugar levels. Interestingly, fenugreek extract also appears to improve testosterone levels and restore the balance between testosterone and cortisol in stressed subjects.

◈ Gymnema

Gymnema (*Gymnema sylvestre*) is a plant used medicinally in India and Southeast Asia for treatment of "sweet urine," or what we refer to in the West as diabetes or hyperglycemia. In ancient Indian texts, gymnema is referred to as "gurmar," which means "sugar killer" in Sanskrit. Gymnema leaves, whether extracted or infused into a tea, suppress glucose absorption and reduce the sensation of sweetness in foods — effects that may deliver important health benefits for individuals who want to reduce blood-sugar levels. *Gymnema sylvestre* leaves contain gymnemic acids, which are known to suppress transport of glucose from the intestine into the bloodstream, and a small protein, gurmar, that can interact with receptors on the tongue to decrease the sensation of sweetness in many foods. Modern scientific methods have isolated at least nine different fractions of gymnemic acids that possess hypoglycemic activity. The effect of gymnema extract on lowering blood levels of glucose, cholesterol, and triglycerides is fairly gradual — typically taking a few days to several weeks. Very high doses of the dried gymnema leaves may even help repair the cellular damage that causes (and is caused by) excessive blood-sugar exposure. Several human studies conducted on gymnema for treatment of diabetes have shown significant reduction in blood glucose, glycosylated hemoglobin (an index of blood-sugar control), and insulin requirements (so insulin therapy could be reduced). Gymnema appears to increase the effectiveness of insulin rather than causing the body to produce more, although the precise mechanism that causes this remains unknown.

◈ Indian Daisy

Indian daisy (*Sphaeranthus indicus*) is a medicinal plant that grows in India, Southeast Asia, and the Philippines. Traditional uses include brewing tea from the flowers as a treatment for diabetes and hyperglycemia (elevated blood sugar). The blood sugar–lowering effect of Indian daisy flower extract is similar to that of insulin, which improves glucose transport from the blood into body cells. The blood sugar–regulating properties of Indian daisy have been demonstrated in studies of isolated cells in animals and humans. In isolated cells, flower extracts are known to stimulate glucose uptake. Feeding diabetic mice, rats, and rabbits Indian-daisy flower reduces elevated blood sugar and returns insulin levels to normal. In humans with moderate abdominal obesity, Indian-daisy flower extract, taken for eight to twelve weeks, has been shown to reduce blood-sugar levels by up to 30 percent and help subjects maintain a tighter control of blood-sugar fluctuations, which helps control appetite and encourage weight loss without significant dietary alterations.

◈ Panax (Asian) Ginseng

Panax ginseng has a more than one-thousand-year history as a folk remedy in China and Korea. In addition to its effects in controlling cortisol as an adaptogen against stress, various animal studies show that Panax ginseng can lower blood sugar, improve glucose utilization, and increase insulin production. A placebo-controlled clinical study showed that Panax ginseng extracts reduce hemoglobin glycosylation and improve glucose tolerance without side effects.

◈ Vanadium

Vanadium is another trace element involved in promoting normal insulin function. A normal diet typically provides about 10 to 30 mcg of vanadium per day. Although no RDA for this element has been established, this amount appears to be adequate for most healthy adults. Vanadium is thought to play a role in the metabolism of carbohydrates and may have functions in cholesterol and blood-lipid metabolism. In diabetics, vanadium supplements may have a positive effect in regulating blood-glucose levels. Food sources of vanadium include seafood, mushrooms, some cereals, and soybeans. Through its insulin-mimetic effect, vanadium is thought to promote glycogen synthesis and help maintain blood-glucose levels. Vanadyl-sulfate supplements have been shown to normalize blood glucose levels and reduce glycosylated hemoglobin levels and can reduce fasting glucose levels by about 20 percent.

◈ Zinc

Zinc is an essential trace mineral for immune function, antioxidant protection, andreproduction. Three out of four people do not get the recommended intakes for zinc. Zinc supplementation is especially important for reducing glycation, because it also promotes normal insulin function. However, to avoid unwanted nutrient interactions, zinc should not be supplemented in high doses (for example, above 45 mg daily) and is best taken in balance with other trace elements, such as copper (2 mg of copper for every 15 mg of zinc).

[vip] SUPPLEMENTS FOR BALANCING STRESS HORMONES

Even though I have saved the "stress" supplements for last, in some ways this aspect can be considered of primary importance to control because of its intimate interactions with the remaining three of the Four Pillars of Health (managing oxidation, controlling inflammation, and stabilizing glucose). Of particular note is to keep in mind that many of the supplements that are effective primarily for balancing stress hormones are also effective as secondary controllers of blood sugar (and thus glycation), free radicals (and thus oxidation), and cytokines (and thus inflammation).

◈ Branched-Chain Amino Acids

The group of amino acids referred to as the "branched-chain amino acids" (BCAAs) comprises three essential amino acids: valine, leucine, and isoleucine. Supplemental levels have been shown to increase endurance, reduce fatigue, improve mental performance, increase energy levels, prevent immune-system suppression, and counteract muscle catabolism following intense exercise.

In numerous studies of athletes, BCAAs have been shown to maintain blood levels of glutamine, an amino acid used as fuel by immune-system cells. During intense exercise and stress, glutamine levels typically fall dramatically, removing the primary fuel source for immune cells and leading to a general suppression of immune-system activity (and an increased risk of infections) following the exercise. By supplementing with glutamine, BCAAs, or both, a person can maintain blood levels of glutamine and thereby avoid suppression of immune-cell activity due to a lack of fuel.

In related studies, BCAA supplements have been shown to help counteract the rise in cortisol and the drop in testosterone that is often seen in endurance athletes undergoing stressful training. In these studies, intense exercise was used as a model for high stress, so the increased cortisol levels and the reduced testosterone levels represented exactly what happens in the average person when they experience a stressful situation at work, at home, or while standing in line at the grocery store.

◈ Ashwagandha

Ashwagandha *(Withania somnifera)* is an herb from India that is sometimes called "Indian ginseng"—not because it is part of the ginseng family but to suggest energy-promoting and antistress benefits that are similar to the ones attributed to the more well-known Asian and Siberian ginsengs. Traditional use of ashwagandha in Indian (Ayurvedic) medicine is to "balance life forces" during stress and aging, similar to the use of cordyceps in restoring

"Qi" (pronounced "chee" and equivalent to the modern description of "vigor") in traditional Chinese medicine and the modern use of many of these "adaptogenic" supplements for restoring vigor. Withanolides are thought to contribute to the calming effects of ashwagandha during periods of stress and may account for the use of ashwagandha as a general tonic during stressful situations (where it is calming and fatigue fighting) and as a treatment for insomnia (where it promotes relaxation).

◈ Beta-sitosterol

Beta-sitosterol is one of hundreds of plant-derived "sterol" compounds that are known to influence cortisol exposure, immune function, and inflammation in the body. Plant oils contain the highest concentration of phytosterols, so nuts and seeds contain fairly high levels, and all fruits and vegetables generally contain some amount of phytosterols. Perhaps the best way to obtain beta-sitosterol is to eat a diet rich in fruits, vegetables, nuts, and seeds (which obviously brings numerous other benefits as well), but beta-sitosterol is available in supplement form as well.

Beta-sitosterol is known to modulate immune function, inflammation, and pain levels through its effects on controlling the production of inflammatory cytokines, and much of this immune/inflammation control appears to be related to an improved interaction of immune cells (which produce inflammatory cytokines) with the adrenal glands (where cortisol is produced). In terms of immune function, beta-sitosterol has been shown to normalize the function of T-helper lymphocytes and natural killer cells following stressful events (such as marathon running), which normally suppress immune-system function. In addition to alleviating much of the postexercise immune suppression that occurs following endurance competitions, beta-sitosterol has also been shown to normalize the ratio of catabolic stress hormones (cortisol) to anabolic (rebuilding) hormones, such as testosterone and DHEA.

◈ Citrus Peel

Citrus peel (*Citrus sinensis*) contains a unique class of flavonoids, known as polymethoxylated flavones (PMFs) — specifically, tangeritin, sinensetin, and nobilitin. The PMFs represent a class of "superflavonoids," extracted from citrus peels, that exhibit approximately threefold potency compared to other flavonoids. PMFs are just what they sound like — flavonoid compounds with extra "methoxy" groups compared to "regular" flavones. Like all flavonoids, the PMFs deliver potent antioxidant and anti-inflammatory activity, but the PMF version is about three times more potent in its ability to restore biochemical balance (and it reduces cortisol levels by about 20 to 30 percent).

Our research group was the first in the world to use PMFs from citrus-peel extract for restoring biochemical balance while also promoting blood-sugar control and weight loss. As part of several research trials, we provided supplements of PMFs (with eurycoma root extract, green-tea catechins, and theanine) to a group of moderately overweight subjects. The PMFs reduced cortisol levels by 20 percent, body weight by 5 percent, body fat by 6 percent, and waist circumference by 8 percent over a period of six weeks. A longer, twelve-week study showed even better results, with additional beneficial effects on reducing cholesterol (by 20 percent), boosting vigor (by 25 percent), reducing fatigue (by 48 percent), and maintaining normal testosterone levels and resting metabolic rate.

◈ Cordyceps

Cordyceps (*Cordyceps sinensis*) is a Chinese mushroom that has been used for centuries to reduce fatigue, increase stamina, improve lung function, and restore "Qi." Traditionally, it was harvested in the spring at elevations above fourteen thousand feet, restricting its availability to the privileged (the emperor and his court). Several studies of cordyceps have shown improvements in lung function, suggesting that athletes may benefit from an increased ability to take up and use oxygen. A handful of studies conducted in Chinese subjects have shown increases in libido (sex drive) and restoration of testosterone levels (from low to normal) following cordyceps supplementation. During stressful events, cortisol levels rise while testosterone levels drop (leading to problems with biochemical balance). Using cordyceps as a way to normalize these suppressed testosterone levels can help modulate the cortisol-to-testosterone ratio within a lower (and healthier) range. At least two chemical constituents—cordycepin (deoxyadenosine) and cordycepic acid (mannitol)—have been identified as the active compounds in improving energy and stamina. Animal studies have shown that feeding with cordyceps increases the level of adenosine triphosphate (ATP) in the liver by 45 to 55 percent, a beneficial effect for boosting energy state and potential for physical and mental performance. Furthermore, mice fed cordyceps and subjected to an extreme low-oxygen environment were able to utilize oxygen more efficiently (30 to 50 percent increase), better tolerate acidosis and hypoxia (lack of oxygen), and live two to three times longer than a control group. In a number of Chinese clinical studies, primarily in elderly patients with fatigue, cordyceps-treated patients reported significant improvements in their levels of fatigue, ability to tolerate cold temperatures, memory and cognitive capacity, and sex drive. Patients with respiratory diseases also reported feeling physically stronger. Recently, a small study presented at the American College of Sports Medicine annual meeting showed that cordyceps significantly increased maximal oxygen uptake and anaerobic threshold, which may lead to improved exercise capacity and resistance to fatigue.

❖ Eurycoma

Eurycoma longifolia, a Malaysian root often called "Malaysian ginseng" for its energy-boosting effects, affords a natural way to bring suboptimal testosterone levels back to within normal ranges. It is also probably the best first-line therapy (before trying synthetic options, such as DHEA supplements or topical/injected testosterone) for anybody suffering from chronic stress. In traditional Malaysian medicine, eurycoma is used as an anti-aging remedy because of its positive effects on energy levels and mental outlook (which are most likely the result of improved biochemical balance and vigor).

Eurycoma contains a group of small peptides (short protein chains), referred to as "eurypeptides," that are known to have effects in improving energy status and sex drive. The "testosterone-boosting" effects of eurycoma appear not to have anything to do with stimulating testosterone synthesis, but rather appear to increase the release rate of "free" testosterone from sex hormone–binding globulin (SHBG). In this way, eurycoma is not so much a testosterone "booster" as a "maintainer" of normal testosterone levels (testosterone that your body has already produced and needs to release to become active). This means that eurycoma is particularly beneficial for individuals with suboptimal testosterone levels, disrupted biochemical balance, and low vigor, including those who are dieting for weight loss, middle-aged individuals (because testosterone drops after age thirty), stressed-out folks, sleep-deprived people, and serious athletes who may be at risk for overtraining.

The vast majority of what we know about eurycoma comes from rodent studies, test-tube binding evaluations, and a handful of open-label human-feeding trials. The test-tube binding studies have shown that eurycoma peptides and related compounds do help release more of the "free" form of testosterone from its binding proteins. The rodent studies have yielded more than a dozen reports of increased energy levels, improved hormonal profiles, and enhanced sex drive. The limited number of human-feeding trials have demonstrated a clear subjective indication of reduced fatigue and heightened energy and mood, as well as a greater sense of well-being in the subjects consuming eurycoma.

Fortunately, a range of specific feeding studies in athletes, dieters, and in stressed and sleep-deprived subjects — who are all under chronic stress and are perhaps the key customers for eurycoma-based products — have been conducted. These studies in "overstressed" subjects used a specific eurycoma root extract prepared with a patented water-extraction and freeze-drying process (developed in collaboration between the government of Malaysia and MIT, the Massachusetts Institute of Technology). In some studies, the patented eurycoma root extract is used alone, and in others, it is blended and balanced with other supplements, such as theanine, citrus PMFs, and green-tea catechins. Overall, these studies found a maintenance of normal testosterone and biochemical balance in supplemented subjects, including dieters (compared to a typical drop in testosterone among nonsupplemented dieters) and cyclists (compared to a typical drop in testosterone in nonsupplemented riders).

For a dieter, it would be expected for cortisol (a catabolic hormone) to rise and testosterone (an anabolic hormone) to drop following several weeks of dieting stress. This change in biochemical balance (cortisol up and testosterone down) is an important cause of the familiar "plateau" that many dieters hit (when weight loss stops) after six to eight weeks on a weight-loss regimen. By maintaining normal testosterone levels, a dieter could expect to also maintain their muscle mass and metabolic rate (versus a drop in both subsequent to lower testosterone levels) and thus continue to lose weight without hitting the dreaded weight-loss plateau.

For an athlete, the same rise in cortisol and drop in testosterone is an early signal of overtraining, a syndrome characterized by reduced performance, increased injury rates, suppressed immune-system activity, increased appetite, moodiness, and weight gain. Obviously, maintenance of normal testosterone levels could prevent some of these overtraining symptoms, as well as help the athlete recover faster and more effectively from daily training bouts.

◈ Ginseng

Ginseng is perhaps the best known of the "adaptogens" (herbs to help the body "adapt" to the biochemical imbalances caused by chronic stress). Several strains of ginseng are available—including Panax ("true") ginseng (also called Korean, or Asian, ginseng), American ginseng, and Siberian ginseng (not a true ginseng; see the next paragraph for more information)—and each type contains some of the same compounds but in slightly different proportions, thus providing slightly different effects in terms of antistress benefits. Numerous animal and human studies have shown that different types of ginseng can increase energy and endurance, improve mental function (learning and maze tests), and improve overall resistance to various stressors, including viruses and bacteria, extreme exercise, and sleep deprivation. Human studies have shown improved immune function and reduced incidence of colds and flu following a month of supplementation with Panax ginseng. In a handful of studies, ginseng supplementation has also provided benefits in mental functioning in volunteers exposed to stress, such as improvements in ability to form abstract thoughts, in reaction times, and in scores on tests of memory and concentration.

Siberian ginseng (*Eleutherococcus senticosus,* or "Eleuthero" for short) is not truly ginseng, but it is a close-enough cousin to deliver some of the same energetic benefits. The Siberian form of ginseng is generally a less-expensive alternative to Panax, or Asian/Korean, ginseng, although it may have more of a stimulatory effect rather than an adaptogenic effect—not necessarily a bad thing if you just need a boost. Often promoted as an athletic performance enhancer, eleuthero may also possess mild to moderate benefits in promoting recovery following intense exercise, perhaps due in part to an enhanced delivery of oxygen to recovering muscles.

The active compounds in ginseng are known as ginsenosides, and most of the top-quality ginseng supplements will be standardized for ginsenoside content. It is thought that the ginsenosides interact within the hypothalamic-pituitary-adrenal (HPA) axis to balance the body's secretion of adrenocorticotropic hormone (ACTH) and cortisol. ACTH has the ability to bind directly to brain cells and can affect a variety of stress-related processes in the body.

❖ Magnolia Bark

Magnolia bark (*Magnolia officinalis*) is a traditional Chinese medicine used since AD 100 for treating "stagnation of Qi" (what we view in Western medicine as low vigor or burnout). Magnolia bark extracts are rich in two biphenol compounds, magnolol and honokiol, both of which are thought to contribute to the primary antistress and cortisol-lowering effects of the plant.

Japanese researchers have determined that the magnolol and honokiol components of magnolia bark extracts are one thousand times more potent than alpha-tocopherol (vitamin E) in their antioxidant activity, thereby helping to balance the "oxidation" Pillar of Health. Other research groups have shown both magnolol and honokiol to possess powerful "mental acuity" benefits via their actions in modulating the activity of various neurotransmitters and related enzymes in the brain (increased choline acetyltransferase activity, inhibition of acetylcholinesterase, and increased acetylcholine release).

Numerous animal studies have demonstrated that honokiol acts as a central-nervous-system depressant at high doses but as an anxiolytic (antianxiety and antistress) agent at lower doses. This means that a small dose of a magnolia bark extract standardized for honokiol content can help to "de-stress" a person, while a larger dose might have the effect of putting you to sleep. When compared to pharmaceutical agents such as Valium (diazepam), honokiol appears to be as effective in its antianxiety activity yet not nearly as powerful in its sedative ability. These results have been demonstrated in at least a half dozen animal studies and suggest that magnolia bark extracts standardized for honokiol content would be an appropriate approach for controlling the detrimental effects of everyday stressors, without the tranquilizing side effects of pharmaceutical agents.

❖ Rhodiola

Rhodiola *(Rhodiola rosea)* is a species of plants from the Arctic mountain regions of Siberia. The root of the plant is used medicinally and is also known as "Arctic root" or "golden root." Rhodiola has been used for centuries to treat cold and flulike symptoms, promote longevity, and increase the body's resistance to physical and mental stresses. It is typically considered to be an adaptogen (like ginseng) and is believed to invigorate the body and mind to increase resistance to a multitude of stresses. The key active constituents in rhodiola are believed to be rosavin, rosarin, rosin, and salidroside.

In one clinical trial, *Rhodiola rosea* extract was effective in reducing or removing symptoms of depression in 65 percent of the patients studied. In another study, twenty-six out of thirty-five men suffering from weak erections or premature ejaculation reported improvements in sexual function following treatment with *Rhodiola rosea* extract for three months. In another study of physicians on nighttime hospital duty, rhodiola supplementation for two weeks resulted in a significant improvement in associative thinking, short-term memory, concentration, and speed of audiovisual perception. An additional study of students undergoing a stressful twenty-day period of exams showed daily rhodiola supplementation alleviated mental fatigue and improved well-being.

Overall, *Rhodiola rosea* extract appears to be valuable as an adaptogen, specifically in increasing the body's ability to deal with a number of psychological and physiological stresses. Of particular value is the theoretical role for rhodiola in increasing the body's ability to take up and utilize oxygen — an effect similar to that of cordyceps (see page 166) — which may explain some of the non-stimulant "energizing" effects attributed to the plant. Rhodiola is often called the "poor-man's cordyceps" because of ancient stories in which Chinese commoners and Tibetan Sherpas used rhodiola for energy because the plants grew wild throughout the country-side, while only the emperor, his immediate family, and his concu-bines were allowed access to the rare cordyceps mushroom.

◈ Theanine

Theanine is an amino acid found in the leaves of green tea *(Ca-mellia sinensis)*. Theanine offers quite different benefits from those imparted by the polyphenol and catechin antioxidants for which green tea is typically consumed. In fact, through the natural production of polyphenols, the tea plant converts theanine into catechins. This means tea leaves harvested during one part of the growing season may be high in catechins (good for antioxidant and anticancer benefits), while leaves harvested during another time of year may be higher in theanine (good for antistress and biochemical-balance effects). Theanine is unique in that it acts as a nonsedating relaxant to help increase the brain's production of alpha waves. This makes theanine extremely effective for com-bating tension, stress, and anxiety, without inducing drowsiness. Clinical studies show that theanine is effective in dosages ranging from 50 to 200 mg per day. A typical cup of green tea is expected to contain approximately 50 mg of theanine.

In addition to being considered a relaxing substance (in adults), theanine has also been shown to provide benefits for improving learning performance (in mice) and promoting con-centration (in students). No adverse side effects are associated with theanine consumption, making it one of the leading natu-ral choices for promoting relaxation without the sedating effects of depressant drugs and herbs. When considering the potential benefits of theanine as an antistress or biochemical-balance sup-plement, it is important to distinguish its nonsedating relaxation benefits from the tranquilizing effects of other relaxing supplements, such as valerian and kava, which are actually mild central-nervous-system depressants.

One of the most distinctive aspects of theanine activity is its ability to increase the brain's output of alpha waves. Alpha waves are one of the four basic brain-wave patterns (delta, theta, alpha, and beta) that can be monitored using an electroencephalogram (EEG). Each wave pattern is associated with a particular oscillating electrical voltage in the brain, and the different brain-wave patterns are associated with different mental states and states of consciousness. Alpha waves, which indicate what we call "relaxed alertness," are nonexistent during deep sleep as well as during states of very high arousal, such as fear or anger. In other words, alpha waves are associated with your highest levels of physical and mental performance; therefore, you want to maximize the amount of time during your waking hours that your brain spends in an alpha state. By increasing the brain's output of alpha waves, theanine can help you "rebalance" your metabolism and your brain-wave patterns as well as help you control anxiety, increase focus and concentration, promote creativity, and improve overall mental and physical performance. Research studies have clearly shown that people who produce more alpha brain waves also have less anxiety, that highly creative people generate more alpha waves when faced with a problem to solve, and that elite athletes tend to produce a burst of alpha waves on the left sides of their brains during their best performances.

11

Putting
Vigor Improvement Practices
to the Test

I t is important to remind yourself from time to time that neither your stress level nor your response to stress is constant.
Instead, there will be periods in your life when you experience
more stress or less stress, just as there will be times when you feel
as if you can withstand stress better and times when it is more difficult to deal with. Accordingly, you need to alter your exercise
patterns, nutrient intake, and supplementation regimen to accom-
modate your exposure to stress. For example, regular exercise and
a balanced diet are always going to be important, but they become
even more so during stressful times. Adhering to your regimen of
dietary supplementation is important every day, but even more so
when you're under periods of elevated stress. Skipping breakfast
during a period of low stress isn't ideal, but it isn't going to kill you.
Skipping that balanced breakfast during a high-stress period sets
yourself up for poor metabolic control and eventual blood-sugar
crashes, surges in appetite, and feelings of fatigue — each of which
will be even more pronounced because of your high-stress profile.

In other words, you almost need to do the opposite of what
most people are tempted to do during high-stress periods — that
is, staying up late to finish work, skipping meals or eating junk

food, and neglecting exercise. Obviously, no one is going to maintain a "perfect" antistress regimen. Nevertheless, if you keep some of the Vigor Improvement Practices (VIPs) in mind and implement them when possible, you'll find it much easier to deal with high-stress periods in your life — and you will enjoy more vigor.

So how can you monitor your response to stress and adjust it in ways that keep you healthy? The best way to start is by evaluating your current stress profile. If you have not yet done so, take the Vigor Self-Test included in the Introduction to get a good baseline gauge of your stress exposure, your vigor, and your degree of biochemical balance. (For your convenience, an additional copy of the test appears in Appendix C, and you can use it to reassess your vigor level as compared to your baseline test.) Are you experiencing higher-than-normal stress levels? If so, then your biochemical balance is likely to be "off," and you need to be especially careful about following steps to restore that biochemical balance and maintain vigor. Are you enjoying an interlude that's relatively stress-free and tranquil? Then perhaps you can relax a bit and take pleasure in the welcome fruits of the healthy lifestyle you've created — and commit to maintaining it.

Wherever you stand after taking the Vigor Self-Test, you can use the questions and results to identify areas in your life that you need to address to regain or maintain vigor. The following sections discuss how to use this test and other tools to enjoy new levels of health.

INCORPORATING VIGOR IMPROVEMENT PRACTICES INTO YOUR LIFE

This book has covered a lot of ground. We've talked about chronic stress, biochemical balance (and imbalance), stress-related diseases, neuroplasticity, and a host of other concepts surrounding vigor. Whew! That's a lot of information to consider — and it all might seem a bit abstract. But as you've been reading this book, you've also learned about numerous practical ideas — especially in the sections on the VIPs. Now it is time to bring those ideas together and apply them. Or as I sometimes say, "Use the VIPs for a VIP": *you!*

As a nutritional biochemist and exercise physiologist studying vigor, I have also become something of a "metabolism coach" over the last decade. By using and teaching the VIP concepts outlined in *The Secret of Vigor,* I've been able to help thousands of clients optimize their own biochemical balance across each of the Four Pillars of Health and achieve the lasting improvements in vigor they have been looking for. You can use those teachings to incorporate the VIPs into your daily life and lifestyle in your own way.

MEASURING YOUR VIGOR VIA THE VIPS

One of the great things about the VIPs is that they are simple and flexible, so you can adapt them to your personal circumstances. Some people will want to jump right into every practice in the book, while others will go more slowly and adopt one or two at a time. Rather than give you "marching orders" for using the VIPs, I am going to recommend two approaches and let you choose whichever works best for you:

❧ A. Monitoring Vigor with the Self-Test

1. Take your Vigor Self-Test (see the Introduction or Appendix C) on Monday morning.

2. For seven days (Monday through Sunday), follow as many of the VIPs as you can (such as getting enough sleep, Interval Walking, taking dietary supplements, etc.).

3. Take your Vigor Self-Test again (using the copy in the Appendix, if you like) on Sunday night to see how you have improved in one short week.

That's it. It couldn't be simpler.

◈ B. Building Vigor by Picking Your Practice

To help you envision the connections between the Four Pillars of Health and the VIPs, I've developed the chart below. You can use this chart to fill in the practices that you want to incorporate into your life. The sample chart gives you an idea of how to do this, and you can use the blank copy of the chart that follows to insert your *own* choices for the VIP that you will try first. Even though each pillar is listed separately, they are all interconnected, so any healthy activity you engage in for one of them will affect all the others, leading to a positive spiral in your vigor. And, even though the example lists only one VIP for each pillar, you can choose to do more than one at any time. So take your time, flip back through the book, and look at the VIP sections in Part III. Underline, highlight, or make a list of the practices that you plan to implement and then write them next to the pillar that you'll be strengthening. You can also take the Vigor Self-Test before you actually begin any of the VIPs you've listed in the chart and then retest yourself again in a few weeks to see how you've progressed.

Your Personal VIPs: Picking Your Practice (Example)

Health Pillar	Vigor Improvement Practice (VIP)
Manage oxidation	Use dietary supplements (See Chapter 10) ...to tap the Anti-Oxidant Network
Control inflammation	Start Interval Training + FlexSkills (See Chapter 9) ...because regular exercise fights inflammation
Stabilize glucose	Apply the Helping-Hand Approach to Eating (See Chapter 8) ...balancing nutrition will help balance blood-sugar levels
Balance stress hormones	Build better sleep habits (See Chapter 7) ...more shut-eye reduces stress and cortisol levels

Your Personal VIPs: Picking Your Practice

(Fill in one or more Vigor Improvement Practices in column two
that you can incorporate into your daily life.)

Health Pillar	Vigor Improvement Practice (VIP)
Manage oxidation	
Control inflammation	
Stabilize glucose	
Balance stress hormones	

ANCIENT WISDOM MEETS MODERN LAB DATA

One of the things that I love most about studying lifestyle interventions (diet and exercise) and traditional remedies (herbal and
dietary supplements) is that researchers often have plenty of "cir-
cumstantial evidence" that they "work," and our studies are frequently confirming (with scientific data) what has already been
observed for decades or centuries. For example, practitioners of
traditional Chinese medicine (TCM) have been using various
herbal remedies for more than three thousand years, but it has only
been in the last two or three decades that any of them have been
"proven" to work by modern scientific investigations. The TCM
practitioners "knew" that certain remedies "worked" for certain

ailments (such as using eurycoma or ginseng to "strengthen the Qi"), but it has taken modern science quite a long time to confirm that these ancient remedies are effective in restoring biochemical balance in the face of many of our own modern diseases.

As a scientist, I find that theories are nice, but evidence is where the rubber meets the road. In the words of many of my colleagues, I want to "see the data" about a particular approach (including the VIPs) before I will believe it works. Based on the data, scientists and health professionals can understand that a given program has a certain degree of likelihood to actually be of benefit to their clients and patients. So over the last handful of years, I have felt very strongly about continuing to put the VIPs "to the test" in order to see if these ideas would really stand up to the harsh reality of restoring biochemical balance and improving vigor in the real world. It all makes "sense" on paper from a biochemical and physiological perspective, but lots of great ideas on paper never made a lick of difference to anyone in the real world.

For close to a decade, my research associates and I have documented the progress of group after group of participants (more than a thousand satisfied participants at last count). The VIPs have been presented in one-week, four-week, six-week, eight-week, and twelve-week versions — and we always set out to recruit as many "hard cases" as we can find. As part of following the VIPs, our participants would meet periodically to talk about how biochemical balance, diet, exercise, and supplements could have an impact on mood, energy, appetite, vigor, and even weight-loss success. In most of our trials, we measured a variety of parameters, including body weight, body fat, metabolic rate, cortisol and testosterone levels, C-reactive protein (CRP), blood glucose, cholesterol values, and stress/mood/vigor levels.

The results were nothing short of dramatic. Virtually every person using the VIPs (more than 90 percent) showed highly significant improvements in feelings of energy, reduced stress/anxiety, and restored vigor (and many lost body weight and body fat as a nice side benefit). Of particular interest with the VIPs is the fact that taking a dietary supplement for controlling stress and improving biochemical balance seemed to help the participants' diet and exercise regimens to "gain traction," compared to the times when they had tried their own versions of diet and exercise alone. In no way does this mean that the supplement was a *substitute* for diet and exercise. However, it suggests strongly that by adding the supplement to their diet and exercise regimens, they were able to reap some additional biochemical balance and thus enjoy greater degrees of vigor. In many ways, the results make perfect "sense," because taking a supplement means that you have additional factors driving you toward biochemical balance (compared to relying on diet and exercise alone).

When we look across the last several years of studying the VIPs with approximately one thousand subjects, we generally find the following "average" results:

- Biochemical balance improves. Cortisol levels drop, and testosterone levels rise, resulting in a rebalancing of the cortisol-to-testosterone (C:T) ratio toward one that favors increased energy, reduced depression, improved mental function, lower tension, and elevated vigor. Our participants generally see a change in this C:T ratio of 15 to 20 percent, and it is one of the major biochemical effects that makes them feel so good, providing them with elevated mood, abundant energy, and clear thinking.

- Vigor, well-being, mood, mental focus, and energy levels increase while depression and tension levels decrease, often by an astonishing amount (15 to 50 percent), due to the restoration of the biochemical balance that has been upset by previous stress exposure.

- Individuals lose about one-half to one pound of fat each week (if they are trying to lose weight via their diet/exercise regimen). I say "fat" instead of just "weight," because it is important to know that our participants are losing the fat and keeping the muscle — meaning they are thinner and healthier, but they maintain their metabolic rate, which helps them keep the weight off. Virtually all the fat loss comes from belly fat, which is logical, because abdominal fat is preferentially stored during periods of elevated stress and upset biochemical balance.

❖ Blood levels of glucose and "bad" cholesterol (LDL) fall by about 20 percent. This is partly due to better eating, partly due to biochemical balance, and partly due to a gradual loss of body fat.

Perhaps the most striking statistic from our studies of the VIPs — even more exciting than the fat loss, the restoration and maintenance of biochemical balance, or even the significant improvement in vigor — is the extremely high compliance rate of more than 90 percent of participants over eight to twelve weeks. The "compliance rate" refers to the percentage of participants who start *and* finish a program or study. In some types of interventions, you may "expect" a low compliance rate, such as weight-loss studies, where we often expect as many as half of all participants to drop out before the study is complete. Having such a high compliance rate for the VIPs is an excellent indicator that these practices are easy enough to follow in "real life" yet effective enough to deliver noticeable and meaningful benefits. Granted, it is not 100 percent — but I'll take a "9 out of 10" success rate every time if I can help bring someone back to a state of life-changing high vigor from a quagmire state of low vigor and burnout.

The data from our various trials of the VIPs have been presented at some of the top nutrition-science conferences in the world, including the International Congress on Nutrition and Fitness, the American College of Nutrition, Experimental Biology (the largest life-sciences conference in the world), the American Society for Nutrition, the American College of Sports Medicine, and the International Society for Sports Nutrition. Attendees at these research conferences generally find that the most interesting feature of the VIPs is not any single aspect of these practices but rather that the synergy between the component parts is so effective when melded into a single and easy-to-follow approach. For example, we've known for years that regular exercise and a balanced diet are the foundations of a healthy lifestyle program. However, what the VIPs show is that by building on the diet/exercise foundation, with specific attention to biochemical balance, the "standard" results, with respect to indices of fatigue, depression, and vigor, can be optimized, much to the delight of the thousands of people who have incorporated the VIPs into their lives.

──────── Scientific Study of the VIPs ────────

The peer-reviewed journal *Progress in Nutrition* has published outlines of two of the clinical trials on the VIPs. I will summarize the text of that manuscript below, and reprints of the article are available at my blog site, www.ShawnTalbott.com.

The idea behind this publication in *Progress in Nutrition* (Volume 12, Number 1, 2010) came from a presentation about "Traditional Medicines as Modern Dietary Supplements" that I was invited to deliver at a scientific conference in Hong Kong. This issue of the *Progress in Nutrition* journal features the proceedings from the 4th International Symposium on Functional Foods entitled, "New Horizons in Chinese Medicines & Health Foods," which took place at the Hong Kong Polytechnic University (sort of like China's version of MIT) on 29–30 October 2009.

It was interesting to participate in the symposium with a broad range of Western scientists and Eastern herbalists. Just as I was speaking about the Western concept of "vigor," other scientists were speaking about the Eastern concept of Qi ("life force") — and we were both speaking about the same concept and using some of the same natural approaches to restore vigor/qi in the face of various types of stress.

The title of the article, "Ancient Wisdom Meets Modern Ailment," highlights the fact that ancient practitioners of traditional medicine used

(cont'd.)

natural approaches for solving health problems and that we can use that same ancient wisdom about herbs and nutrients to counteract some of today's most debilitating conditions (such as chronic stress, burnout, depression, chronic fatigue, mental fog, and many others).

The objective in the studies outlined in the *Progress in Nutrition* paper was to assess changes in vigor, mood state, and biochemical balance in response to implementing the VIPs. The VIPs included the same modest lifestyle interventions outlined in this book, including the Helping-Hand Approach to Eating, the Interval Walking and FlexSkill exercises, the recommendation to strive for eight hours of nightly sleep, and a combination of herbal supplements. The combination of supplements used in both the studies outlined in the *Progress in Nutrition* paper included four components: eurycoma, citrus PMFs, green-tea catechins, and theanine. Each of these is also used in traditional Asian medicine to improve "life force" and well-being in stressed or fatigued individuals.

The *Progress in Nutrition* paper reported on eighty-two subjects, all displaying moderate levels of psychological stress. We specifically recruit volunteers for our studies who self-report at least a "moderate" level of psychological stress. In these studies, we measured biochemical-balance parameters (cortisol and testosterone), mood-state parameters, and related subscales, such as vigor, fatigue, and depression, using the Profile of Mood States (POMS) psychological survey before and after the intervention (either eight weeks or twelve weeks following, depending on the study).

Our results were dramatic and fairly well replicated between the two different studies. Compared to preintervention values (before starting the VIPs), measurements taken after eight or twelve weeks of following the VIPs indicated significant changes in:

- biochemical balance (15 to 19 percent improvement in the ratio between cortisol and testosterone)
- vigor (27 to 29 percent increase)
- fatigue (41 to 48 percent reduction)
- depression (40 to 52 percent reduction)
- global mood state (20 to 22 percent increase in this "overall" measurement of well-being)

Our overall conclusion from these studies was that "these data indicate that factors that are typically disrupted during periods of chronic stress (metabolic hormone profile and psychological mood state) may be positively and significantly impacted by modest changes in diet, exercise, and supplementation patterns that mirror those commonly used in traditional Asian medicine." These results, and many more like them using the same VIP interventions to restore biochemical balance and improve vigor under different types of stress, have proven to me over and over again the accuracy of the idea that I started with at the beginning of this book—that "biochemistry drives our behaviors" and is responsible for a great deal of how we feel and how we perform on a daily basis. In our studies, we repeatedly see how stress can disrupt numerous aspects of our biochemical balance and how those disruptions lead to low vigor and eventually to burnout and outright disease. But we also see how restoring that biochemical balance across each of the Four Pillars of Health, using sleep/stress management, diet, exercise, and supplements, can help beat burnout and restore vigor.

CONCLUDING WORDS

Even your dear old grandmother knew some of the basic steps underlying biochemical balance and high vigor: Get enough sleep, eat right, and exercise. Yes, it is a tired, old mantra, but these three steps are probably the most effective tools available for combating stress and raising levels of wellness. Stress researchers around the world, from Yale to Sweden to the University of California, have shown over and over that the best way of "managing" stress, from a physical and a psychological perspective, is to adhere to a handful of basic tenets of good health promotion, such as the following:

1. *Move it!* It doesn't even really need to be "exercise," as long as you're out there moving your body from point A to point B — and often (daily) — and for about an hour per day (though not necessarily all at the same time).

2. *Stop eating* before you're stuffed. Use the "80 percent rule" so that you eat until you're not hungry (80 percent full).

3. *Find an outlet for your stress.* Everyone has stress that needs to be released. The stress is toxic, and it is stronger than you — get rid of it.

4. *Get a life.* Cultures with the longest life spans and the highest "happiness quotients" tend to have well-developed social networks that emphasize making family and friends a priority, living a spiritual life, and encouraging individuals to have a "purpose" in life.

5. *Relax.* Sleep. Be lazy (every once in a while).

Decades of scientific research show that stress — and failure to adhere to the five basic tenets listed above — does a lot of "bad things" to people. The loss of vigor and most "modern" diseases are stress-related and directly result from the biochemical imbalances that stress creates.

Yet as I sit here writing this book at the beginning of the second decade of the twenty-first century, I'm also marveling at the research breakthroughs that have given us so much more insight into the impact of chronic stress, the importance of biochemical balance, and the need to strengthen the Four Pillars of Health. We now know that we can use the VIPs to bring about meaningful changes in how the body responds to stress and how people perform and feel every day. I hope that, by this point in the book, you've come to the conclusion that everyone needs to "do something" about their chronic stress exposure, and I also hope that I've made a compelling-enough case for you to give the VIPs a try.

Restoring your vigor will truly change your life — and when it does, I hope that you will be motivated to share what you have learned in this book to help others change their lives as well.

APPENDIX A | *Recipes*

Here is an entire week of delicious breakfast, lunch, and dinner recipes — seven of each meal. Each meal has been created to incorporate as many aspects of the Four Pillars of Health as possible and help you use the right ingredients to restore biochemical balance (by managing oxidation, controlling inflammation, stabilizing glucose, and balancing stress hormones).

Feel free to mix and match them each day to your own tastes — and when you can't treat yourself to one of these outstanding meals, keep the Helping Hand "rules" in mind and combine your carbs/fats/proteins according to the guidelines in Chapter 8. Remember, this is a basic set of recipes — people who need gluten-free, vegan, or dairy-free recipes should be able to develop some of their own over time. Others may be concerned about the high fat content in some recipes, but that is intended to deliver an effective dose of anti-inflammation fatty acids and antioxidant nutrients — exactly in-line with the recommendations underlying the Four Pillars concepts.

These recipes come to us specially crafted by New York City chef Michael Saccone. Since age fourteen, Michael Saccone has worked for many restaurants, catering companies, and clubs. Most notably, he apprenticed at George Perrier's Le Bec Fin in Philadelphia, worked at the four-star Le Cirque in New York City, and worked privately for several high-profile celebrity clients. As a private chef, he has gained experience in health-conscious cooking. Currently he is employed by Maury Povich at his eponymous television program and in the family home. Michael is also the owner of City Chef Corporation, which produces prepared side dishes that accompany meats, poultry, and seafood for Manhattan's top specialty markets. Michael resides in New York City with his wife, Adrienne, and two young children, Catherine and Elizabeth.

Bon appétit!

Breakfast

Oatmeal Blueberry Pancakes with Almond Butter

PER SERVING: CALORIES (KCAL) 502 — SODIUM (MG) 827 — FAT (G) 28 —
CARBOHYDRATES (G) 49 — SATURATED FAT (G) 11 — FIBER (G) 6 —
CHOLESTEROL (MG) 177 — SUGAR (G) 20 — PROTEIN (G) 14 — CALCIUM (MG) 366

Pancakes made with oat, some flour, buttermilk, and dense with blueberries, topped with butter creamed with sweetened almond paste. (Serves 4)

½ cup all-purpose flour
1 cup rolled oats
½ tablespoon baking powder
½ tablespoon baking soda
½ teaspoon salt
1½ cups buttermilk or milk

2 tablespoons peanut oil
3 eggs, separated
1 pint blueberries
½ stick soft butter
2 ounces almond paste or
marzipan

1. Grind almond paste into butter in a bowl with the back of a spoon or in a food processor until well incorporated and smooth. Set aside.
2. Sift together dry ingredients. In large bowl, beat yolks and gradually add peanut oil and then buttermilk. Beat egg whites to soft peaks.
3. Start to heat grill pan or skillet over medium heat.
4. Gradually stir dry ingredients into yolk mixture, stopping when ingredients are just combined. Fold in beaten whites, starting with just a little to lighten the mixture, and then add the rest. Fold in blueberries.
5. Test skillet with a drop of water (it should sizzle, not instantly evaporate) and add about a teaspoon of butter to pan, swirling it to coat entire surface. When butter is sizzling but not yet brown, ladle out pancakes. The pancakes should look firm and have well-formed dimples when you flip them. Brown flipped side and serve hot with almond butter spread over the cakes, like you would spread it on toast.

Breakfast

Smoked Salmon and Arugula Omelet

PER SERVING: CALORIES (KCAL) 298 — SODIUM (MG) 1,929 — FAT (G) 19 —
CARBOHYDRATES (G) 6 — SATURATED FAT (G) 5 — FIBER (G) 1 —
CHOLESTEROL (MG) 437 — SUGAR (G) 3 — PROTEIN (G) 24 — CALCIUM (MG) 102

Omelet stuffed with smoked salmon and peppery arugula sautéed
with Bermuda onion. (Makes 1 large omelet for 2)

Olive oil
1 small Bermuda onion
1 bunch arugula
½ tablespoon capers
1 pinch red pepper flakes

4 large eggs
1 tablespoon milk
½ teaspoon salt
4 ounces smoked salmon

1. Skin onion, remove core, cut in half, and slice into ⅛-inch slices.
2. Place sauté pan over medium heat, add about ½ tablespoon olive
   oil and onions, and start to cook until soft, flipping occasionally,
   about 4 minutes.
3. Trim stems from arugula, wash in large bowl with cold water,
   remove leaves, and shake off water.
4. Turn up heat on onions, add a little more olive oil if necessary,
   and add red pepper flakes, capers, and arugula, with a pinch of
   salt. Cook greens, tossing frequently, until they wilt, about a
   minute. Place mixture into a bowl with a strainer, wipe pan with
   a paper towel, and return to heat, reducing flame to medium.
5. Scramble eggs with milk and salt. Add about another ½ tablespoon olive oil to pan and swirl around. When a test drop of
   water sputters, add eggs to pan, let eggs start to set a few seconds,
   and stir gently with a spatula, allowing eggs to set a little again
   before repeating stir. When eggs are about two-thirds cooked,
   reduce heat to low, and allow omelet to take shape. Place greens
   mixture up the center from 12 o'clock to 6 o'clock and top with
   salmon. When eggs are done, flip one side over and slide omelet
   onto serving dish.

Sweet Breakfast Biscuits and Gingered Prunes

PER SERVING: CALORIES (KCAL) 454 — SODIUM (MG) 281 — FAT (G) 13 —
CARBOHYDRATES (G) 78 — SATURATED FAT (G) 7 — FIBER (G) 5 —
CHOLESTEROL (MG) 77 — SUGAR (G) 33 — PROTEIN (G) 7 — CALCIUM (MG) 204

Breakfast "cookies" made with toasted millet and eaten with stewed gingered prunes. (Serves 4)

For Biscuits:

¼ cup hulled millet seeds	⅓ cup sugar
⅔ cup water	4 tablespoons butter
1 cup all-purpose flour	1 egg
2 teaspoons baking powder	1 teaspoon vanilla

1. Toast millet in pan over medium-low heat until golden and starting to pop. Add water, cover pan, and reduce heat to low, cooking until liquid is gone, about 15 minutes.
2. Cream butter and sugar, and add egg and vanilla. Sift flour and baking powder together into butter mixture. Stir in millet.
3. Place spoonsful of mixture on sheet pan lightly coated with nonstick spray or parchment paper. Bake for about 12 minutes, or until golden. Let cool on sheet.

For Prunes:

1 cup pitted prunes
1 piece ginger, 1 inch
Water

1. Slice ginger in half, and add to small saucepan with prunes. Add enough water to just cover, and bring to a gentle simmer. Cook for 20 minutes, transfer to a bowl, and refrigerate until cool and thick syrup forms, about 3 hours.

Breakfast

Crunchy Yogurt Parfait

PER SERVING: CALORIES (KCAL) 369 — SODIUM (MG) 141 — FAT (G) 5 —
CARBOHYDRATES (G) 76 — SATURATED FAT (G) 0 — FIBER (G) 9 —
CHOLESTEROL (MG) 0 — SUGAR (G) 47 — PROTEIN (G) 7 — CALCIUM (MG) 142

Parfait made with alternating layers of berries, vanilla yogurt, and granola. (Serves 2)

½ pint blueberries
½ pint raspberries
2 tablespoons honey

2 granola bars, crumbled
1 cup low-fat vanilla yogurt

1. In separate bowls, place berries and 1 tablespoon honey for each. Stir to coat well and place in refrigerator for 1 hour, gently stirring every 15 minutes.
2. In 2 parfait cups or tall glasses, place alternating layers starting with yogurt, sprinkle with granola, blueberries, yogurt, granola, raspberries, yogurt, and a final sprinkle of granola.

Buckwheat Hazelnut Muffins

PER SERVING: CALORIES (KCAL) 349 — SODIUM (MG) 303 — FAT (G) 20 —
CARBOHYDRATES (G) 34 — SATURATED FAT (G) 6 — FIBER (G) 4 —
CHOLESTEROL (MG) 50 — SUGAR (G) 16 — PROTEIN (G) 7 — CALCIUM (MG) 66

One of my personal breakfast favorites, these muffins are made with buckwheat flour and flavored with hazelnut, orange, and raisins. (Makes 12)

¾ cup raisins	1 teaspoon salt
1 orange	¼ teaspoon ground cloves
1 cup blanched hazelnuts	6 tablespoons butter
1¼ cups all-purpose flour	½ cup sugar
1 cup buckwheat flour	2 eggs
1 tablespoon baking powder	½ cup sour cream
½ tablespoon baking soda	

1. Preheat oven to 375 degrees Fahrenheit.
2. In a microwave safe bowl, zest and juice orange, add raisins, cover with plastic, and microwave for 30 seconds. Let sit to allow raisins to plump.
3. Toast hazelnuts in one layer on a sheet pan in oven (about 10 to 15 minutes).
4. Sift dry ingredients together.
5. Cream butter and sugar until fluffy and add 1 egg at a time, letting first egg fully incorporate before adding the second. Add sour cream and raisin mixture. Stir in dry ingredients until just uniformly mixed. Fold in hazelnuts.
6. Fill paper-lined muffin tin three-fourths full for each muffin. Bake about 15 minutes or until golden. Let cool in pan.

Breakfast

Parmesan Florentine Eggs

PER SERVING: CALORIES (KCAL) 391 — SODIUM (MG) 1,149 — FAT (G) 20 —
CARBOHYDRATES (G) 32 — SATURATED FAT (G) 4 — FIBER (G) 10 —
CHOLESTEROL (MG) 373 — SUGAR (G) 6 — PROTEIN (G) 24 — CALCIUM (MG) 429

Whole-grain toast slice topped with sautéed spinach, red peppers, and sliced olives and finished with gratinéed eggs. (Serves 2)

2 bunches leaf spinach	4 eggs
1 sweet red pepper	1 teaspoon vinegar
¼ cup pitted Alfonzo olives	3 ounces Parmesan cheese, grated
1 small shallot	2 slices seven-grain bread
Olive oil	

1. Trim stems from spinach and place in large bowl filled with cold water. Lift leaves out and place in colander. Drain water, rinse bowl of sand, and repeat.
2. Cut pepper in half. Remove stem, seeds, and ribs and slice halves into ⅛-inch pieces.
3. Drain olives and cut into quarters. Peel shallot and mince.
4. Fill shallow pan with water and bring to a simmer. Add vinegar and crack eggs, gently releasing them into water as close to the surface as possible. Poach eggs to desired doneness.
5. While eggs poach, heat sauté pan over high heat, and add about ½ tablespoon olive oil and peppers. Sauté until soft, add shallot, and cook another 30 seconds, tossing continuously. Add spinach and toss until wilted. Season with salt and pepper. Transfer to a bowl with a strainer in it and allow to drain.
6. Toast bread on sheet pan under broiler, flipping to toast both sides. Place half the spinach mixture on each slice, covering bread completely. Next place two poached eggs on top of each bed of spinach mixture. Sprinkle with cheese and slide pan under the broiler again until cheese browns, about 30 seconds.

Garden Frittata

PER SERVING: CALORIES (KCAL) 232 — SODIUM (MG) 266 — FAT (G) 10 —
CARBOHYDRATES (G) 20 — SATURATED FAT (G) 3 — FIBER (G) 2 —
CHOLESTEROL (MG) 372 — SUGAR (G) 3 — PROTEIN (G) 15 — CALCIUM (MG) 82

Frittata crowded with broccoli, tomato, chard, and red onion, bound with a bit of whole-wheat pasta. (Serves 4)

8 large eggs
2 ounces dry soba noodles
1 cup broccoli florets
1 bunch Swiss chard, trimmed
and washed
1 tomato

1 yellow pepper
1 red onion
1 clove garlic, minced
⅛ teaspoon red pepper flakes
Salt
Olive oil

1. Preheat oven to 350 degrees Fahrenheit.
2. Bring medium pot of water to a boil. Add enough salt so it almost tastes like the ocean. Fill a large bowl with ice water.
3. Cook broccoli in boiling salted water until tender, about 2 to 3 minutes. Remove from water with slotted spoon or spider and plunge directly into ice water. Repeat with Swiss chard. Drain and set aside. Cook soba in salt water, drain, and set aside.
4. Remove stem end from tomato and cut in half, east to west. With fingers, poke out seeds while lightly squeezing tomato half. Chop tomato into ½-inch pieces.
5. Cut pepper in half and remove stem, seeds, and ribs. Slice into ⅛-inch slices.
6. Cut onion in half, skin, remove stem, slice into ⅛-inch slices.
7. Scramble the eggs.
8. Heat 9-inch sauté pan over medium heat (nonstick works best). Add about ½ tablespoon olive oil and onions. Sauté about 3 minutes and add peppers. When peppers are soft, add garlic, cook another 30 seconds, then add tomato, broccoli, Swiss chard, and soba noodles. Season aggressively with salt and stir in beaten eggs. Turn heat to low and let cook about 2 minutes. Slide pan into oven and bake until set, about 30 minutes.
9. When done, slide frittata out of pan and onto serving platter. Cut into quarters and serve.

Curry Chicken Salad

PER SERVING: CALORIES (KCAL) 484 — SODIUM (MG) 169 — FAT (G) 23 —
CARBOHYDRATES (G) 60 — SATURATED FAT (G) 4 — FIBER (G) 13 —
CHOLESTEROL (MG) 30 — SUGAR (G) 41 — PROTEIN (G) 16 — CALCIUM (MG) 211

Tender Boston lettuce and curried chicken sweetened with green apples, raisins, and walnuts. (Serves 4)

2 pounds chicken thighs	¾ cup golden raisins
½ onion chopped into 4 quarters	½ cup walnuts
1 celery stalk chopped into 4 sections	2 heads Boston lettuce
1 carrot chopped into 4 sections	½ cup low-fat yogurt
1 bay leaf	¼ cup mayonnaise
4 green apples	1 tablespoon curry powder
	Salt and pepper

1. Remove skin from chicken thighs, place thighs in medium saucepan, and fill with water to a level 2 inches over meat. Place pan over medium-high flame and bring to gentle simmer. Skim all the scum and fat that come to the surface, and add onion, celery, carrot, and bay leaf. Simmer for 45 minutes, skimming from time to time. Turn off heat and transfer to bowl. Allow chicken to cool in broth.
2. Remove meat from thigh bones in large pieces and remove vein. Dice meat into ½-inch cubes. Strain broth and freeze it for future use.
3. Dice 2 of the apples into ¼-inch cubes, leaving on skin. Mix with walnuts and raisins.
4. Whisk yogurt, mayonnaise, and curry until smooth. Fold in apple–nut mixture. Fold in chicken and add salt and pepper to taste. Let sit covered in refrigerator.
5. Remove tough leaves and core from lettuce and wash leaves in large bowl of cold water. Spin dry. Arrange beds of lettuce on 4 plates. Slice remaining 2 green apples in half, remove cores, and slice halves into ¼-inch slices. Arrange slices on lettuce and distribute chicken salad in mounds over the apple slices and lettuce.

Gazpacho with Avocado Cream

PER SERVING: CALORIES (KCAL) 299 — SODIUM (MG) 764 — FAT (G) 17 —
CARBOHYDRATES (G) 34 — SATURATED FAT (G) 2 — FIBER (G) 13 —
CHOLESTEROL (MG) 0 — SUGAR (G) 16 — PROTEIN (G) 7 — CALCIUM (MG) 124

Cold vegetable soup thick with celery, cucumber, sweet and hot peppers, scallions, carrots, and tomato, flavored with extra virgin olive oil, red wine vinegar, and herbs. Served with hearty grain bread. (Serves 2)

1 cucumber	*1 teaspoon Worcestershire sauce*
1 carrot	*1½ tablespoons red-wine vinegar*
2 ribs celery	*Dash hot sauce*
1 tomato	*Salt and freshly ground*
1 green pepper	*black pepper*
1 jalapeño pepper	*1 ripe avocado*
4 scallions	*½ lime*
⅛ cup chopped parsley	*Salt and pepper*
1 can V8 juice, 8 ounces	*Extra virgin olive oil*
1 can tomato juice, 8 ounces	

1. Peel carrot and cucumber. Remove seeds from cucumber by cutting lengthwise and scooping with spoon. Cut tomato in half, east to west, and remove seeds and core at top. Cut peppers in half and remove seeds, stems, and ribs. Finely dice peppers and cucumber and set aside in large bowl.
2. Roughly chop carrot, scallion, and celery. Pulse in food processor until finely chopped but not starting to lose liquid, and add to bowl. Repeat with tomato. Add parsley to bowl, as well as juices, Worcestershire, vinegar, and hot sauce. Salt and pepper to taste. Chill well.
3. Cut avocado in half, remove pit, and scoop from skin into processor. Add juice of ½ lime and process until smooth. Salt and pepper to taste.
4. Ladle soup into chilled bowls and dollop avocado in center. Lace top with quick swirl of olive oil. Serve with hearty bread.

Turkey Tabbouleh

PER SERVING: CALORIES (KCAL) 492 — SODIUM (MG) 704 — FAT (G) 28 —
CARBOHYDRATES (G) 36 — SATURATED FAT (G) 4 — FIBER (G) 8 —
CHOLESTEROL (MG) 81 — SUGAR (G) 3 — PROTEIN (G) 28 — CALCIUM (MG) 42

Bulgur grain mixed with diced turkey breast, tomatoes, olives, scallions, and chopped parsley, finished with lemon and olive oil. Served on a bed of shredded lettuce. (Serves 4)

1 cup bulgur grain
1 cup boiling water
1 teaspoon salt
2 tomatoes
½ cup pitted Kalamata olives
1 bunch scallions
2 bunches flat-leaf parsley

1 large lemon
¼ cup olive oil
Salt and pepper
1 pound roast turkey breast
1 small head iceberg lettuce, shredded

1. Place bulgur and salt in a medium bowl, add boiling water, and cover with plastic wrap. Let soak until liquid is absorbed, about 35 minutes.
2. Cut tomatoes east-west, remove core at top, and chop into ¼-inch pieces. Place in medium bowl and set aside. Trim and clean scallion in cold water and chop, then add to tomatoes. Wash parsley in large bowl of cold water, shake or spin dry, and chop, avoiding stems. Slice olives and add to tomatoes with parsley. Dice turkey into ½-inch cubes and add to vegetables.
3. Remove plastic from bowl of bulgur and fluff grain with fork. Squeeze lemon juice and add to bulgur with olive oil, continuing to fluff with fork. Add vegetables and turkey by fluffing in as well, and add salt and freshly ground pepper to taste.
4. Place lettuce on 4 plates and spoon tabbouleh over lettuce.

Greek Dinner Salad

PER SERVING: CALORIES (KCAL) 530 — SODIUM (MG) 1,080 — FAT (G) 42 —
CARBOHYDRATES (G) 19 — SATURATED FAT (G) 9 — FIBER (G) 6 —
CHOLESTEROL (MG) 67 — SUGAR (G) 7 — PROTEIN (G) 22 — CALCIUM (MG) 270

Romaine and spinach garnished with cucumbers, tomato, olive, onion, and feta cheese. Topped with marinated chicken breast brushed with an herb vinaigrette. (Serves 4)

2 boneless, skinless chicken breasts,
approximately 4 ounces each
2 lemons
½ cup olive oil
1 teaspoon dried oregano
1 small clove garlic, minced
¼ teaspoon freshly ground
black pepper

1 teaspoon salt
1 head romaine lettuce
1 bunch leaf spinach
1 cucumber
2 tomatoes
½ red onion
½ cup Kalamata olives
8 ounces feta cheese

1. With the fine side of a box grater, grate the yellow part of skin of 1 lemon. Place in jar or food-storage container with lid. Add juice from lemons, oregano, salt, pepper, garlic, and olive oil. Shake.
2. Cut each chicken breast lengthwise to separate into two thinner pieces. Trim off cartilage, fat, and tenders. Place each piece between plastic wrap and pound evenly to about ½-inch thickness. Place pieces in pan where they do not overlap and pour ⅓ dressing over them, turning to coat. Cover with plastic and place in refrigerator.
3. Trim and clean lettuce and spinach in bowl of cold water. Lift leaves out and repeat washing with fresh cold water. Chop leaves into ¾-inch pieces and spin dry.
4. Peel and seed cucumber and slice halves into ¼-inch slices. Remove top core of tomatoes and cut 8 wedges from each tomato. Slice onion half as thinly as possible.
5. Pat chicken dry with paper towel, season with salt and pepper, and rub on some olive oil. Place in pan under broiler and cook through, flipping breasts when halfway done. Remove from oven and brush breasts with some of the vinaigrette.

6. Toss leaves with remaining vinaigrette and adjust salt and ground pepper to taste. Create a bed of leaves on each plate, arrange 4 tomato wedges on each, and equally distribute the cucumber, onion, olives, and feta cheese. Top each with a chicken breast half.

Classic Club Broccoli Salad

PER SERVING: CALORIES (KCAL) 369 — SODIUM (MG) 311 — FAT (G) 30 —
CARBOHYDRATES (G) 16 — SATURATED FAT (G) 4 — FIBER (G) 8 —
CHOLESTEROL (MG) 13 — SUGAR (G) 5 — PROTEIN (G) 14 — CALCIUM (MG) 150

Crisp blanched broccoli tossed with bacon, currants, and smoked almonds. (Serves 2)

1 head broccoli	*⅓ cup mayonnaise*
Salt	*1 tablespoon distilled vinegar*
4 slices bacon	*1 tablespoon sugar*
4 ounces smoked almonds	*Salt and freshly ground*
¼ cup currants	*black pepper*

1. Fill a large bowl with ice water and set aside. Cut florets off into bite-size pieces. Bring medium pot of water to a boil and add salt until it almost tastes like the ocean. Drop broccoli in water and cook 1 minute. Lift out broccoli with slotted spoon and plunge into bowl of ice water. When broccoli is cool, drain and place in colander to dry.
2. Cook bacon in skillet or microwave until crisp. Crumble bacon and mix in bowl with smoked almonds and currants.
3. Whisk mayonnaise, vinegar, and sugar. Fold in broccoli and nut mixture. Add salt and freshly ground pepper to taste.

Asian Shrimp Salad

PER SERVING: CALORIES (KCAL) 250 — SODIUM (MG) 190 — FAT (G) 8 —
CARBOHYDRATES (G) 18 — SATURATED FAT (G) 1 — FIBER (G) 3 —
CHOLESTEROL (MG) 172 — SUGAR (G) 11 — PROTEIN (G) 27 — CALCIUM (MG) 111

Shrimp, sweet peppers, scallions, grapes, cilantro, and crushed peanuts dressed with a sweet and sour sauce. (Serves 4)

1 pound peeled raw shrimp
1 teaspoon Chinese five-spice
powder
1 teaspoon salt
½ tablespoon peanut oil
1 red pepper
1 bunch scallions
1 carrot

1 bunch watercress
⅛ cup chopped cilantro
Juice of 1 lime
1 teaspoon fish sauce
1 tablespoon rice vinegar
1 teaspoon sugar
½ pound seedless grapes
¼ cup peanuts, crushed

1. Heat skillet over medium-high heat and test with water drop for
   fast sputter. Add peanut oil, sprinkle shrimp with five-spice
   powder and salt, and sear in skillet on each side until firm and
   cooked (times vary on size of shrimp, but about 1 minute and 30
   seconds each side should do). Set aside cooked shrimp to cool.
2. Wash scallions and slice thinly on a diagonal in 1-inch lengths.
   Core, seed, and remove ribs from pepper and slice thinly into
   1-inch lengths. Trim end of watercress, chop into 1-inch lengths,
   wash in cold water, and spin dry. Combine all in large bowl.
3. Whisk lime juice, fish sauce, vinegar, and sugar together. Pour
   over vegetables and toss. Place mixture on platter, arrange
   shrimp on top, and sprinkle with crushed peanuts. Garnish with
   grapes.

Tuna Niçoise Salad

PER SERVING: CALORIES (KCAL) 474 — SODIUM (MG) 536 — FAT (G) 23 —
CARBOHYDRATES (G) 47 — SATURATED FAT (G) 3 — FIBER (G) 12 —
CHOLESTEROL (MG) 100 — SUGAR (G) 7 — PROTEIN (G) 23 — CALCIUM (MG) 156

Green beans, tomato, hard-boiled egg, Niçoise olives, and tuna on Bibb lettuce with Dijon vinaigrette. (Serves 2)

2 eggs	2 heads Bibb lettuce
1 tomato	1 teaspoon Dijon mustard
4 ounces French green beans	½ clove garlic, minced
2 ounces Niçoise olives	Juice of 1 lemon
¼ red onion	1 teaspoon sugar
4 small red or yellow potatoes	¼ cup olive oil
1 teaspoon salt	Pinch dried thyme

1 can tuna, packed in olive oil, 6 ounces

1. Place eggs in small pan and cover with water; bring to simmer over medium-high heat. Cover and turn off heat. After 7 minutes, remove eggs and plunge into ice water.
2. Place potatoes in small pan with enough water to cover and add salt. Bring to simmer over medium-high heat and cook until knife can easily penetrate. Cool.
3. Bring medium pan of water to boil, with enough salt added to make it taste almost like the ocean. Trim beans and cook 2 minutes. Remove with slotted spoon and plunge into ice water. When beans are cool, drain them.
4. Prepare vinaigrette by combining mustard, sugar, thyme, and garlic in a small bowl with a whisk. Add olive oil, a drop at a time at first, and whisk into an emulsion. Gradually add oil in a steady, thin stream while continuously whisking. Season with salt and freshly ground pepper.
5. Trim and wash Bibb lettuce and spin dry. Peel eggs and cut into quarters. Cut small potatoes into quarters. Slice onion as thinly as possible. Core and cut tomato into wedges. Place lettuce on platter in bed and arrange vegetables and eggs around parameter of platter. Place drained tuna in center and garnish with olives. Serve vinaigrette on the side.

Pesto Bluefish

PER SERVING: CALORIES (KCAL) 750 — SODIUM (MG) 726 — FAT (G) 41 —
CARBOHYDRATES (G) 38 — SATURATED FAT (G) 10 — FIBER (G) 10 —
CHOLESTEROL (MG) 132 — SUGAR (G) 8 — PROTEIN (G) 58 — CALCIUM (MG) 507

Basil-crusted bluefish with broccoli and tomato, sautéed with shallot and white wine. (Serves 2)

12 ounces bluefish filet
2 slices white bread, crust removed and diced
1 bunch basil, cleaned and chopped
¼ cup pine nuts
2 ounces Parmesan, grated
1 tablespoon olive oil
Salt and pepper

Olive oil
1 bunch broccoli, florets cut into bite-size pieces
1 tomato, seeded and chopped
Juice of 1 lemon
1 shallot, peeled and minced
1 clove garlic, thinly sliced
¼ cup dry white wine
½ tablespoon butter

1. Preheat oven to 400 degrees Fahrenheit.
2. Add salt to medium pot of water until it almost tastes like the ocean; heat to a boil over high flame.
3. In food processor, grind bread into fine crumbs and set aside in bowl. Pulse basil and pine nuts to break them down, stopping every 3 or 4 pulses to scrape sides with spatula. When mixture becomes fairly smooth, add Parmesan and blend. Add olive oil in a steady stream while machine is running. Fold mixture into crumbs and season with salt and pepper to taste.
4. Cut filet into two pieces. With back of spoon, smear pesto on fish surface in an even ¼-inch layer. Place filets in buttered pan, crust side up, and add a few tablespoons water. Bake in oven until cooked through and top is slightly brown, about 12 minutes.
5. While fish cooks, heat large sauté pan over medium-high heat. Add broccoli to boiling salted water. Pour about ½ tablespoon oil into sauté pan along with garlic and shallot, stirring to avoid burning, and heat for about 1 minute. Add tomatoes and cook another minute. Add wine and allow liquid to reduce about 1 minute. Remove broccoli from boiling water with a slotted spoon and place broccoli directly into sauté pan with tomato

mixture. Add lemon juice and butter, reduce heat to medium, and stir slowly and continuously until creamy — do not overheat or butter will break down. Remove pan from heat and adjust seasoning with salt and freshly ground pepper. Divide mixture between 2 plates and top with fish.

Dinner

Soba Primavera

PER SERVING: CALORIES (KCAL) 649 — SODIUM (MG) 1,332 — FAT (G) 34 —
CARBOHYDRATES (G) 61 — SATURATED FAT (G) 8 — FIBER (G) 2 — CHOLESTEROL
(MG) 37 — SUGAR (G) 2 — PROTEIN (G) 29 — CALCIUM (MG) 573

Japanese buckwheat noodles tossed with sautéed greens, portobello mushrooms, grape tomatoes, olives, garlic, and shallots, and finished with Parmesan and chives. (Serves 2)

2 bundles soba noodles, about	*clean and diced*
4 ounces	*½ cup grape tomatoes, halved*
1 tablespoon salt	*½ cup olives, sliced*
Olive oil	*1 clove garlic, minced*
1 bunch kale, trimmed and	*1 shallot, peeled and thinly sliced*
washed	*3 ounces Parmesan, grated*
1 portobello mushroom, wiped	*⅓ bunch chives, chopped*

1. Bring medium pot of salted water to boil. Add soba and cook according to time indicated on the package. Reserve 1 cup cooking water and drain noodles.
2. Heat large sauté pan over medium-high heat and add about 1 tablespoon olive oil and mushroom. Allow to cook until released liquid has dried and add garlic, shallot, olives, and tomatoes. Season with salt and pepper and cook another 2 minutes. Put vegetables into bowl, wipe pan with paper towel, add ½ tablespoon olive oil, and heat until almost smoking. Add kale and sauté about 30 seconds to coat with oil, then add about ⅓ cup reserved noodle water to pan and cover with lid. Cook until kale is tender, stirring occasionally, about 3 minutes. Add vegetables, noodles, and Parmesan and toss all ingredients together. Add a bit more reserved noodle water if dish starts to get dry. Divide between 2 plates and sprinkle chives on top.

Mediterranean Salmon

PER SERVING: CALORIES (KCAL) 610 — SODIUM (MG) 229 — FAT (G) 36 —
CARBOHYDRATES (G) 29 — SATURATED FAT (G) 12 — FIBER (G) 12 —
CHOLESTEROL (MG) 137 — SUGAR (G) 13 — PROTEIN (G) 44 — CALCIUM (MG) 105

Broiled salmon with spicy ratatouille (stewed eggplant, yellow and green squash, red peppers). (Serves 2)

1 center salmon filet, 12 ounces
2 tablespoons butter
½ tablespoon chopped fresh parsley
½ teaspoon fresh lemon zest
Salt and freshly ground pepper
Olive oil
1 small to medium yellow squash

1 small to medium zucchini
1 red pepper
1 medium eggplant
½ red onion
2 cloves garlic, minced
Pinch red pepper flakes
Pinch dried thyme
2 tablespoons tomato paste

1. Cut squash, zucchini, and eggplant into ½-inch cubes by cutting along the side of the vegetable ⅓-inch deep to produce "sheets," and cut each sheet into cubes. Discard the seedy cores. Dice onion into ½-inch pieces.
2. Mix butter with parsley and lemon. Add salt and pepper to taste.
3. Heat medium-sized sauté pan over medium-high heat with about ¼ tablespoon olive oil and add yellow squash. Season squash with salt and pepper and lower heat to medium, making sure squash is cooked through but not mushy. Set aside in medium saucepan. Repeat with zucchini, eggplant, and red pepper. Sauté onion until translucent over medium heat and add pepper flakes, thyme, and garlic. Cook 1 minute and add tomato paste, mixing so the paste comes into as much contact with sauté pan surface as possible. Fold other vegetables into saucepan and set over very low heat. Adjust seasoning with salt and freshly ground pepper.
4. Heat broiler on high. Cut fish into 2 pieces, season with salt and freshly ground pepper, and place on foil-lined sheet pan rubbed with a little olive oil. Place pan a few inches from broiler and cook fish through on one side, allowing to brown a bit on top.
5. Distribute ratatouille between two plates and place salmon on top; top each piece of hot fish with compound butter.

Dinner

Mackerel Escabeche

PER SERVING: CALORIES (KCAL) 700 — SODIUM (MG) 725 — FAT (G) 37 —
CARBOHYDRATES (G) 47 — SATURATED FAT (G) 7 — FIBER (G) 12 —
CHOLESTEROL (MG) 119 — SUGAR (G) 8 — PROTEIN (G) 48 — CALCIUM (MG) 436

Spanish mackerel sautéed and then marinated in a mixture of onions, peppers, and sherry vinegar. Serve with spinach and wheat-berry sauté. (Serves 2)

Olive oil	*½ tablespoon sugar*
1 mackerel filet, 12 ounces	*Pinch red pepper*
Flour for dredging	*½ cup wheat berries*
1 small red onion, thinly sliced	*1 cup water*
1 yellow or red pepper, sliced	*2 teaspoons salt*
¾ cup sherry vinegar	*2 bunches leafy spinach, trimmed*
½ cup water	*and washed*
2 cloves garlic, sliced thin	*Salt and freshly ground pepper*

1. Heat wheat berries, salt, and water in small saucepan over medium-high heat. When water starts to simmer, cover with lid and reduce heat to lowest setting. Wheat berries should cook in about 35 minutes; test them occasionally until they reach the ideal level of slight chewiness, and add more water if necessary.
2. Heat medium-sized skillet over medium-high heat. Cut fish into 2 even pieces, season with salt and pepper, and dredge in flour. Add about ½ tablespoon olive oil and sauté fish on both sides until cooked through. Remove fish from pan and set aside.
3. Add ½ tablespoon olive oil to pan, along with onions and peppers. Cook over medium heat for about 3 minutes or until peppers start to soften. Drain excess oil from pan and add garlic and pepper flakes. Stir over medium-high heat for 30 seconds, deglaze with water and vinegar, and add sugar. When sugar dissolves and onions are soft, pour over fish. Let sit.
4. Wipe sauté pan with paper towel and return to high heat. Add about ½ tablespoon olive oil and heat to nearly smoking. Add spinach and generous pinch of salt, then sauté. When spinach is wilted, add cooked wheat berries. Spinach is finished when tender, about 1 minute more. Divide among 2 plates. Serve with marinated fish.

Spicy Grilled Shrimp and Quinoa

PER SERVING: CALORIES (KCAL) 664 — SODIUM (MG) 365 — FAT (G) 28 —
CARBOHYDRATES (G) 50 — SATURATED FAT (G) 4 — FIBER (G) 13 —
CHOLESTEROL (MG) 344 — SUGAR (G) 4 — PROTEIN (G) 56 — CALCIUM (MG) 226

Shrimp dusted with spice and grilled, served with quinoa salad with avocado, cucumber, cilantro, and lime. (Serves 2)

¾ pound large shrimp, peeled	1 cucumber
1 teaspoon cumin	3 scallions
1 teaspoon salt	1 avocado
½ teaspoon paprika	1 lime
¼ teaspoon ground black pepper	¼ cup chopped cilantro
½ cup quinoa	1 tablespoon olive oil
1½ cups water	Salt and pepper
½ teaspoon salt	Romaine lettuce
	Lime wedges

1. Mix cumin, salt, paprika, and black pepper.
2. Rinse quinoa with cold water. Place in pan with 1½ cups water and salt. Bring to boil, cover, and reduce heat to low. Quinoa will be ready in 12 to 15 minutes. Remove lid and fluff with fork.
3. Peel cucumber, slice in half lengthwise, and remove seeds with spoon. Dice halves into ¼-inch pieces.
4. Clean scallions and slice into thin crosswise, green and white parts, but discard roots at base.
5. Cut avocado in half around pit. Pull apart, remove pit, and separate skin from halves with large spoon. Dice avocado halves into ¼-inch pieces and immediately toss with lime juice. Add to cooked quinoa, along with cucumber, scallions, and cilantro. Drizzle in olive oil and add salt and freshly ground pepper to taste.
6. Heat large skillet over medium-high heat, add about ½ tablespoon olive oil, and swirl it around in pan. Toss shrimp with spice mixture and add shrimp to pan, one at a time, gently pressing shrimp on pan surface. Allow to sear about 1½ minutes or until shrimp has a light-pink color, flip, and finish cooking. Line two plates with romaine, place half quinoa mixture in center of each plate, and arrange shrimp around salad. Serve with additional lime wedges.

Dinner

Steak with Cream Spinach and Millet Croquettes

PER SERVING: CALORIES (KCAL) 635 — SODIUM (MG) 619 — FAT (G) 24 —
CARBOHYDRATES (G) 34 — SATURATED FAT (G) 8 — FIBER (G) 10 —
CHOLESTEROL (MG) 163 — SUGAR (G) 2 — PROTEIN (G) 72 — CALCIUM (MG) 563

Your favorite steak, simply prepared and combined with a healthy dose of spinach and millet. (Serves 4)

*Steak of your choice, prepared via
desired method
4 bunches curly spinach, washed
and trimmed
¼ cup cream
Salt and pepper
½ cup millet
2 cups water
3 scallions, washed and chopped*

*1 clove garlic, minced
1 red pepper, finely diced
1 teaspoon Worcestershire sauce
Dash Tabasco sauce
1 egg, scrambled
2 ounces Parmesan, grated
¼ cup all-purpose flour
Olive oil*

1. Fill large pot with water and bring to boil. Add enough salt so water tastes almost like the ocean. Add spinach and cook until tender, about 2 minutes after water returns to boil. Remove spinach and plunge into cold water. Squeeze spinach dry and put into processor. Pulse until spinach breaks up evenly, scraping down sides. When spinach is fairly uniform, run processor continuously and add cream in a steady stream. Add salt and freshly ground pepper to taste.
2. Bring millet and water to a boil, cover, and simmer until liquid is gone, about 30 minutes. Set aside and let rest.
3. In a sauté pan, add about ½ tablespoon olive oil and sauté red pepper with scallion until soft. Add garlic and cook 30 seconds more. Fluff millet with fork and add scallion mixture, Tabasco sauce, Worcestershire, egg, Parmesan, and flour. Add salt and pepper to taste. Form mixture into balls the size of golf balls and flatten into disks. Heat skillet with olive oil and cook until brown. Flip and put into oven for 12 minutes or until cooked through. Serve on platter with reheated creamed spinach and steaks.

Dinner

Southern Stuffed Pork Chops and Red Flannel Hash

PER SERVING: CALORIES (KCAL) 542 — SODIUM (MG) 640 — FAT (G) 23 —
CARBOHYDRATES (G) 30 — SATURATED FAT (G) 9 — FIBER (G) 5 —
CHOLESTEROL (MG) 123 — SUGAR (G) 10 — PROTEIN (G) 44 — CALCIUM (MG) 119

Pork chops stuffed with Swiss chard and served with hash made from sweet potatoes, beets, and bacon. (Serves 4)

4 pork chops, 6 ounces each	½ tablespoon cornstarch
1 bunch Swiss chard	1 tablespoon water
Olive oil	2 sweet potatoes
2 red onions chopped, divided	2 medium beets
1 clove garlic, minced	4 slices bacon
2 tablespoons white vinegar	¼ cup sour cream
Dash Tabasco sauce	2 tablespoons Dijon mustard
¼ cup cream	⅛ cup chopped parsley
2 tablespoons bulgur	Salt and pepper
¾ cup white wine	

1. Preheat oven to 375 degrees Fahrenheit.
2. Wash and dry beets and sweet potatoes, prick all around with knife, rub with olive oil, season with salt and pepper, and wrap in foil. Place in oven and cook until knife is easily inserted, about an hour.
3. Bring medium-sized pan filled with water to boil over high heat. Trim and wash Swiss chard in large bowl of cold water, shake dry, and chop into 2-inch pieces. Add enough salt to boiling water so it almost tastes like the ocean and add Swiss chard. Cook until tender, about 4 to 6 minutes. Drain chard from pot and plunge into ice cold water.
4. Warm sauté pan over medium heat and add ½ tablespoon olive oil and half the onions. Cook until onions are translucent. Add garlic and turn up heat to medium high. Cook garlic about 30 seconds, stirring, and add Swiss chard. Cook another minute and add vinegar. After vinegar reduces (about a minute), add cream and bulgur. Stir until thickened, about 3 minutes, and set aside to cool.

5. With a small knife, cut into center of the side opposite the bone of each pork chop. Once knife is inserted, pivot it carefully from side to side, avoiding breaking all the way through, to make a pocket. Stuff each pocket with one-fourth of stuffing, and close pocket with toothpicks.

6. Heat ½ tablespoon olive oil in sauté pan just large enough for the chops. Season chops with salt and pepper and sear on each side. Remove chops from pan and deglaze with wine. Reduce by half, turn off heat, return chops to pan, and cover pan with foil. Place in oven and cook to desired doneness, being careful not to dry out chops (start checking after 20 minutes).

7. Peel cooled sweet potatoes and beets. Dice into ¼-inch pieces and mix in with parsley, mustard, and sour cream. Add salt and pepper to taste. Heat bacon in skillet until crisp and crumble into mixture. Pour mixture into pan with bacon drippings, spread evenly, and cook over medium-high heat until crisp. Flip and crisp on other side.

8. Remove chops from pan and return to medium-high heat. Combine cornstarch with water to make a slurry and whisk into juices to make gravy. Gravy will thicken when it reaches boiling. Cook another minute and adjust seasoning.

9. Divide hash and pork chops among 4 plates and serve with gravy.

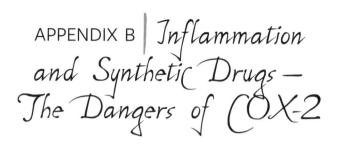

APPENDIX B | Inflammation and Synthetic Drugs — The Dangers of COX-2

The discussion in Chapter 4 focuses on a variety of options for naturally controlling inflammation, while it also points out some of the problems with using synthetic drugs, such as those that inhibit the COX-2 (cyclo-oxygenase-2) enzyme. This special section provides greater detail on the dangers associated with these drugs.

The Cox-2 Catastrophe

In February 2005 the Food and Drug Administration (FDA) convened an advisory meeting to look into the debacle surrounding the elevated risk of heart attack and stroke associated with use of drugs in the "COX-2" class of pain relievers. As mentioned earlier, this class of medications includes Merck's Vioxx (removed from the market) and Pfizer's Celebrex (still on the market), as well as a third drug, Bextra (pulled from the market by Pfizer following the "suggestion" from the FDA to do so). All are under growing scrutiny for causing a variety of heart problems. To defend itself against Vioxx claims, Merck set aside a legal war chest of $675 million — an amount that might sound substantial, but pales in comparison to the $21.1 billion that another drug company, Wyeth, has paid to settle claims against its "fen-phen" weight-loss drug and the $1.11 billion that Bayer has paid on claims against its dangerous cholesterol drug Baycol. With twenty million people having taken Vioxx at some time since its launch in 1999, the legal costs for Merck could be staggering.

To make matters even worse (giving you a headache if you didn't already have one) is the news that naproxen (the drug you may know as Aleve), and indeed the whole class of drugs in the category of NSAIDs, has also been implicated in a variety of adverse side effects from heart problems to gastrointestinal and liver problems (see table below). In addition, the painkiller acetaminophen (Tylenol), which is not strictly in the same chemical class as the other NSAIDs, has recently been linked to severe liver toxicity, lung problems (associated with reduced levels of glutathione, an antioxidant), and high blood pressure. It seems that using synthetic drugs to control pain and inflammation is risky business no matter which drug you choose.

Pain-Reliever Roulette

OTC = over the counter; Rx = prescription

Drug	Brands	OTC/ Rx	Sales (2008*)	Pros	Cons
Aceta-minophen	Tylenol	OTC	$780m	Reduces pain, easy on stomach	Does not reduce inflammation, may cause liver damage and lung damage, increases blood pressure
Aspirin	Bayer, Anacin	OTC	$280m	Reduces pain and inflammation, protects heart	Thins blood, can cause stomach ulcers, strokes, and kidney failure
Celecoxib	Cele-brex	Rx	$2.6b	Reduces pain, easy on stomach	Increased risk of heart attack and stroke
Ibuprofen	Advil, Motrin	OTC	$700m	Reduces pain and inflammation, lower risk of stomach problems compared to aspirin	Ulcers and other gastrointestinal damage
Naproxen	Aleve	OTC	$270m	Reduces pain, especially in joints, long-lasting effect	Gastrointestinal damage, increased risk of heart attack and stroke
Oxycodone	Oxy-Contin	Rx	$1.9b	Reduces chronic pain	Addictive narcotic, patients can develop tolerance

(cont'd.)

Pain-Reliever Roulette (cont'd.)

OTC = over the counter; Rx = prescription

Drug	Brands	OTC/ Rx	Sales (2008*)	Pros	Cons
Rofecoxib	Vioxx	Rx	$1.8b	Reduces pain, easy on stomach	Doubles risk of heart attack and stroke
Valdecoxib	Bextra	Rx	$940m	Reduces pain	Gastrointestinal damage, increased risk of heart attack and stroke

* The 2008 stats are the most recent figures that provide a reasonable comparison across the different drug categories (OTC versus prescription).

COX-2 Inhibitors—The "Miracle" That Wasn't

Why are COX-2 drugs different from other painkillers? Aspirin and older painkillers like ibuprofen block the COX-1 *and* COX-2 enzymes that are involved in pain and inflammation (COX-2) but that are also involved in normal function of the stomach, kidneys, and other tissues (COX-1). Vioxx, Celebrex, and Bextra are unique, because they only block the COX-2 enzyme (a good and bad situation). Blocking COX-1 can reduce pain and actually improve heart health, but it also leads to gastrointestinal problems, such as stomach ulcers (causing about seventeen thousand deaths — *deaths!* — each year from GI bleeds induced by such drugs as naproxen and ibuprofen). *If a dietary supplement or herbal extract caused seventeen thousand deaths per year — or ever — you could bet that a natural-products industry would no longer exist — but with drugs, this is apparently an acceptable outcome.* The thought was that by leaving COX-1 alone and only blocking COX-2, you could obtain pain relief (in arthritic joints, for example) without the gut damage. This is indeed a boon for those chronic-pain patients who do not find adequate relief from arthritis and other conditions with the older pain relievers. However, clinical trials have *not* shown Vioxx, Celebrex, or Bextra to be any more effective in managing pain than the older and cheaper painkillers — but differences can exist between patients that allow one drug to work better than another.

Although I'm in full support of the rights of patients and physicians to assess their own risk/benefit tolerances when it comes to drug choices and other self-care decisions, newer evidence is suggesting that consumers and doctors may not have been given all the necessary information on which to base their decisions about COX-2-inhibiting drugs. For example, COX-2 inhibitors may suppress the formation of certain proteins that are needed to reduce blood clotting (thus increasing clot formation and heart-attack risk). On this issue, I mostly agree with the FDA that this class of drugs should be prescribed only to the very small group of patients who can draw enough unique pain/GI benefits to outweigh the increased risks to heart health and not to the millions of consumers who were duped into believing that these "wonder" drugs were perfectly safe. I'm not alone in this regard — many medical experts felt back in 1999 that the COX-2 inhibitor drugs simply did not offer an appreciable benefit-to-risk ratio and thus should not have been approved (or perhaps should have been approved *only* for those arthritis patients at highest risk for ulcers and other GI problems).

APPENDIX C | *The Vigor Self-Test*

- For each question, write your score in the corresponding column.
- For each answer of "Never/No"—give yourself zero (0) points.
- For each answer of "Occasionally"—give yourself one (1) point.
- For each answer of "Frequently/Yes"—give yourself two (2) points.
- For the last question (#16)—SUBTRACT 1 point for each of the words that closely describes how you have been feeling during the past TWO WEEKS.

Question—"How Often Do You..."

1. ...experience stressful situations? _____
2. ...feel tired or fatigued? _____
3. ...get fewer than eight hours of sleep? _____
4. ...feel anxious/depressed? _____
5. ...feel overwhelmed or confused? _____
6. ...have a low sex drive? _____
7. ...put on weight around the belly? _____
8. ...diet to lose weight? _____
9. ...attempt to control your body weight? _____
10. ...pay close attention to the foods you eat? _____
11. ...crave carbohydrates (sweets or breads)? _____
12. ...experience problems concentrating? _____
13. ...experience tension headaches? _____
14. ...experience digestive problems or heartburn? _____
15. ...get sick or catch colds/flu? _____

Scoring (add above numbers #1–#15)   **points**   _____

16. …feel lively, active, energetic, cheerful, alert, full of pep, carefree, or vigorous (one point for each, 0–8 total)?   _____

Total (subtract total for #16 from total for #1–#15) **points**   _____

Vigor Index

0–5 points   **High Vigor** (Excellent Biochemical Balance)
You are cool as a cucumber and have either a very low level of stress or a tremendous ability to deal effectively with incoming stressors. Keep doing what you're doing!

6–10 points   **Average Vigor** (Acceptable Biochemical Balance)
You may be suffering from an overexposure to stress or an overactive stress response, and you are at moderate risk of being chronically out of biochemical balance, leading to reduced vigor. You should incorporate anti-stress strategies into your lifestyle whenever possible to maintain (and improve) your biochemical balance and vigor. But don't stress out about it!

Greater than 10 points   **Low Vigor** (OUT of Biochemical Balance)
The bad news is that you're almost definitely suffering from an overactive stress response, chronically disrupted biochemical balance, and a low state of vigor—and you need to take immediate steps to regain control. The good news is that you're not alone—literally millions of people are in the same situation.

References

The Secret of Vigor is heavily researched and documented; therefore, the References, which are only a partial list of the works consulted in writing *The Secret of Vigor,* are very lengthy. In an effort to have the book be reasonably priced and to conserve paper, the References can be found online at www.SecretofVigor.com.

Resources

There are vast amounts of scientific and medical information concerning the details underlying each of the biochemical and psychological processes I discuss in this book — far too much information to even summarize here. For interested readers, I invite you to more fully explore these intricacies at some of my educational websites and some of the many excellent books that delve more deeply into the science of dietary supplements, stress physiology, and positive psychology.

Educational Websites

The Author's Personal Blog (www.ShawnTalbott.com)

SupplementWatch — a guide to helping consumers and health professionals make smart decisions about choosing and using dietary supplements (www.SupplementWatch.com)

Wisdom of Balance — an online resource for helping people achieve "balance" in their bodies for optimal health, wellness, and vigor (www.WisdomofBalance.com)

Killer at Large — an award-winning documentary film exploring the causes and solutions underlying the American obesity epidemic (www.KilleratLarge.com)

Cortisol Control and the Beauty Connection — *The All-Natural Inside-Out Approach to Reversing Wrinkles, Preventing Acne, And Improving Skin Tone* (www.CortisolControl.com)

Natural Solutions for Pain-Free Living — *Flexible Joints, Strong Bones, and Ache-Free Muscles for Life* (www.PainFreeLivingBook.com)

The Cortisol Connection — *Why Stress Makes You Fat and Ruins Your Health* (www.CortisolConnection.com)

The Cortisol Connection Diet — *The Breakthrough Program to Control Stress and Lose Weight* (www.CortisolConnectionDiet.com)

Recommended Reading on Dietary Supplements

Talbott, Shawn M. *A Guide to Understanding Dietary Supplements: Magic Bullets or Modern Snake Oil.* New York: Haworth Press — Taylor & Francis Group, 2003.

Talbott, Shawn M., and Kerry Hughes. *The Health Professional's Guide to Dietary Supplements.* New York: Lippincott, William & Wilkins, 2006.

Recommended Reading on Positive Psychology and Brain Plasticity

Begley, Sharon. *Train Your Mind, Change Your Brain: How a New Science Reveals Our Extraordinary Potential to Transform Ourselves.* New York: Ballantine Books, 2007.

Ben-Shahar, Tal. *Happier: Learn the Secrets to Daily Joy and Lasting Fulfillment.* New York: McGraw-Hill, 2007.

Csikszentmihalyi, Mihaly. *Finding Flow: The Psychology of Engagement in Everyday Life.* New York: Basic Books, 1998.

Doidge, Norman. *The Brain That Changes Itself: Stories of Personal Triumph from the Frontiers of Brain Science.* New York: Penguin, 2007.

Gilbert, Daniel. *Stumbling on Happiness.* New York: Vintage, 2007.

Lyubmirsky, Sonja. *The How of Happiness: A Scientific Approach to Getting The Life You Want.* New York: Penguin Press, 2008.

Seligman, Martin. *Authentic Happiness.* New York: Free Press, 2004.

Recommended Reading on Stress Physiology

Lee, Roberta A. *The SuperStress Solution.* New York: Random House, 2010.

Sapolsky, Robert M. *The Trouble with Testosterone: And Other Essays on the Biology of the Human Predicament.* New York: Scribner, 1998.

———. *Why Zebras Don't Get Ulcers.* New York: Holt, 2010.

Index

Boldface page numbers refer to recipes located in the text.

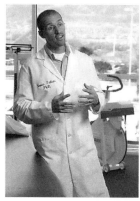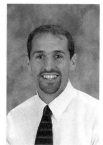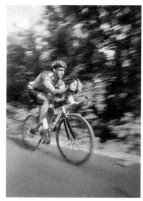

About the Author

Dr. Shawn Talbott received dual bachelor's degrees in Sports Medicine (BS) and Fitness Management (BA) from Marietta College, his master's degree (MS) in Exercise Science from the University of Massachusetts, and his PhD in Nutritional Biochemistry from Rutgers University. His research is primarily focused on metabolism, weight loss, sports nutrition, and human performance. Dr. Talbott has also undertaken postgraduate studies in Entrepreneurship at the Massachusetts Institute of Technology's Sloan School of Business as part of MIT's curriculum with the Entrepreneur's Organization (EO) and the highly selective, three-year Entrepreneurial Masters Program (EMP).

Dr. Talbott is the recipient of a dozen competitive research awards and has published more than two hundred articles on nutrition, health, and fitness. He has served as a nutrition consultant and educator for elite-level athletes in a variety of sports, including professional triathletes, members of the Utah Jazz (NBA basketball), the U.S. Ski and Snowboard Association during the 2002 Winter Olympic Games, and the Performance Enhancement Team (PET) for the U.S. Track and Field Association, and the U.S. Olympic Training Centers.

As an athlete himself, Dr. Talbott has competed at the national and international level in rowing (as part of the U.S. National Team Development Program) and triathlon (completing more than one hundred marathons and triathlons, including fourteen at the Ironman distance).

Dr. Talbott has reviewed articles and served on the editorial boards for several scientific journals, including the *Journal of Dietary Supplements*, the *American Journal of Preventive Medicine*, the *International Journal of Sports Nutrition*, *Current Topics in Nutraceutical Research*, and the *Journal of Nutraceuticals, Functional & Medical Foods*.

Dr. Talbott is the former director of the University of Utah Nutrition Clinic and taught as an associate clinical professor in the Department of Nutrition, where he received the Outstanding Instructor Award in 2004. At the University of Utah, Dr. Talbott received competitive teaching grants to develop on-campus and online versions of the nation's first full-semester graduate-level course on the research and development of dietary supplements. He is a Fellow of the American College of Sports Medicine (ACSM), the American College of Nutrition (ACN), and the American Institute of Stress (AIS), and he holds professional memberships in the American Society for Nutrition (ASN) and the International Society for Sports Nutrition (ISSN).

Currently, Dr. Talbott maintains an active nutrition-research program near Salt Lake City, Utah, where he serves as research director at SupplementWatch (a health education company) and as chief scientific officer for Wicked Fast Sports Nutrition (a product research and development company).

Dr. Talbott's most recent projects include the recent book *The Secret of Vigor* (about the detrimental health effects of chronic stress) and *Killer at Large — Why Obesity Is America's Greatest Threat* (an award-winning, feature-length documentary film exploring the startling details underlying the American obesity epidemic).

Dr. Talbott's Books/Films:

- *Killer At Large — Why Obesity Is America's Greatest Threat* (Disinformation Co., 2009)

- *The Cortisol Connection: Why Stress Makes You Fat and Ruins Your Health* — 2nd Edition (Hunter House, 2007)

- *The Health Professionals Guide to Dietary Supplements* — with Kerry Hughes, M.Sc. (Lippincott, Williams & Wilkins, 2007)

- *Cortisol Control and the Beauty Connection: The All-Natural, Inside-Out Approach to Reversing Wrinkles, Preventing Acne, and Improving Skin Tone* (Hunter House, 2007)

- *Natural Solutions for Pain-Free Living: Flexible Joints, Strong Bones & Ache-Free Muscles for Life* (Currant Book, 2006)

- *The Cortisol Connection: Why Stress Makes You Fat and Ruins Your Health* (Hunter House, 2002).

- *The Cortisol Connection Diet: The Breakthrough Program to Control Stress and Lose Weight* (Hunter House, 2004). Selected as featured book for Amazon.com's "Connect" program for "top authors."

- *A Guide to Understanding Dietary Supplements* (Haworth Press, 2003). Selected as "Outstanding Academic Text" by *Choice* — The Journal of University Research Librarians.